# What to Do When Your Child Isn't Talking

# What to Do When Your Child Isn't Talking

Expert Strategies to Help Your Baby
or Toddler Talk, Overcome Speech Delay,
and Build Language Skills for Life

## NICOLA LATHEY and TRACEY BLAKE

sheldon PRESS

First published in the United States by
The Experiment, LLC in 2023
Originally published as *Small Talk: How to Develop Your Child's Language Skills from Birth to Age Four* by The Experiment, LLC, in 2014

First published in Great Britain by Sheldon Press in 2023
An imprint of John Murray Press
A division of Hodder & Stoughton Ltd,
An Hachette UK company

1

Text design by Beth Bugler

A CIP catalogue record for this title is available from the British Library

Trade Paperback ISBN 978 1 399 80976 4
eBook ISBN 978 1 399 80977 1

Typeset in ITC Galliard Std.

Printed and bound in Great Britain by Clays Ltd, Elcograf S.p.A.

John Murray Press policy is to use papers that are natural, renewable and recyclable products and made from wood grown in sustainable forests. The logging and manufacturing processes are expected to conform to the environmental regulations of the country of origin.

John Murray Press
Carmelite House
50 Victoria Embankment
London EC4Y 0DZ

www.sheldonpress.co.uk

*For our children—Jess, Minnie, and Monty*

# Contents

# Introduction: How this book can help your child talk

For the past twenty-four years, I've been fortunate enough to have my dream job—I am a children's speech and language therapist (the US equivalent of which is a speech-language pathologist, or SLP). My work has taken me to child development centers as far afield as Australia, India, Sri Lanka, and Vietnam, but now I am based in Oxford, England, where I run my own private practice, The Owl Centre.

I specialize in working with children under the age of five and have helped patients with all sorts of speech, language, and communication problems—from babies who aren't yet babbling to toddlers who are more interested in Thomas the Tank Engine than talking to children whose speech has been severely affected by their dummy addiction.

When I wrote the first edition of this book, at the time titled *Small Talk*, I would never have predicted what I am seeing now: growing numbers of children whose speech has been severely impacted and delayed by the COVID-19 pandemic. Sadly, the lengthy lockdowns, constant wearing of masks (meaning babies couldn't watch people's mouths move to copy them), school closures, and lack of playgroups and opportunities to socialize with others have taken a huge toll on those vital early years of children's speech and language development. Those early years are when the brain builds neural pathways to learn new skills; for instance, pathways from the jaw, lips, and tongue establish the foundations of talking.

Of course we can't blame this all on COVID. The huge increase in our smartphone use is another large contributing factor. Every time I go downtown or on the school run, I see a parent who is scrolling through their phone ignoring their child, missing a great opportunity to be talking and interacting with their baby or toddler about what their child can see around them. It's almost as if parents have forgotten that they need to talk to their babies to help them speak—and keep chatting with them once they can. Hopefully this book will help turn that tide the other way.

I want to provide support and strategies to worried parents whose children find talking challenging. This updated edition covers all of your key concerns. Whatever questions you may have about your child's language development, I am here to answer them. I always think the worst point in time for a parent is when you have a niggle at the back of your mind, perhaps for some time, and you're not sure whether you should or shouldn't be worried. Or perhaps you are definitely worried and not sure what you can do to help.

In this book, we cover topics that include: Is my child autistic or are they suffering from speech delay? Why can't my 18-month-old say "Mummy" when all her peers can? Maybe you're wondering why your child constantly shouts or why you can't understand a word your child says. Does your friend boast that her baby has mastered 100 words, while yours only knows 10?

Whatever your reason for picking up this book, it has been written to reassure and help you take positive action, because when it comes to encouraging communication, you really are your child's best resource.

# THIS BOOK CAN HELP YOU . . .

## Easily identify speech concerns and use expert strategies to overcome them

*What to Do When Your Child Isn't Talking* takes a super practical problem–solution approach. Clear chapter headings will help you identify what's going on with your child's communication and focus on the problem. In each chapter I'll explain what you can do to help solve the issue by encouraging or resetting the natural stages of language development with fun games and activities. I want to teach you how you can build language skills for life so you can bring up a child who is confident, social, curious, and happy.

## Know what stage your child has reached and how to help them to the next milestone

I'm constantly quizzed about speech, language, and communication development—by friends, the checkout lady in our local store who knows what I do for a living, and even strangers on the street who have seen me coming out of my clinic. Almost without exception, they want reassurance that what their child is doing is "normal" for their age, or they ask about what might be considered "a problem" or a "delay." I put these words in scare quotes for a reason: We all have perfectly imperfect children who are individuals and who develop at their own rate.

If your child doesn't seem to be speaking like their peers, you might be relaxed or frantically worried. I've seen children who can hold conversations at 18 months, while others of the same age can barely say a recognizable sound. Both are perfectly acceptable and therefore "normal."

But given the exceptional circumstances we've been living in and the devastating impact the pandemic has had on speech development, the concerns that our children have fallen behind the usual milestones are more common than ever. Speech delay has, in effect, become the new normal, so it's even harder for parents to identify whether their child has a different issue that needs to be addressed. This book will help you to work out if there's an issue and to take positive action, so you can stop worrying!

## Have a calmer, happier home

If a child struggles to communicate and seems to be getting annoyed, it may be because there is a gap between their current cognitive ability and their level of speech; they don't yet have the language capability to express what they want. This can result in frustration and temper tantrums as they struggle to verbalize their thoughts. So, the earlier your child can communicate—whether it's to tell you that they want to play with the red car, would like a drink, or are feeling too hot—the less frustrated and the calmer they will be.

Of course, a child's inability to communicate what they want or need isn't only frustrating for the child. Parents can feel helpless when their child struggles to tell them something and they simply cannot understand what it is. By helping them to become confident talkers you will help to reduce the frustrations of both you and your child, so you will feel calmer, too!

## Give your child a head start at school

A study at the University of Kansas showed that the greater the number of words children heard from their parents or caregivers before the age of three, the higher their IQ and the better they did in school.[1] They found that children with a positive communication environment went on to achieve higher scores on tests of language, reading, and math when they entered school. The project is the first large-scale study to examine the impact of children's early environment (before they are two) on their language. The findings emphasize that what parents do with their children, even before they have started to talk, can help prepare them for school and lifelong learning. Professor Sue Roulstone, director of the Speech and Language Therapy Research Unit for North Bristol Trust, says, "The main message is that, as parents, we can have a big impact on how our children learn to talk, and the better our children are talking by the age of two years, the better they will do when they start school."

*What to Do When Your Child Isn't Talking* will help you and your child unlock and unblock the magic of communication. The way that you communicate and engage with your child will affect not only how they interact with you but also how they approach the world, express themselves, learn, pick up social skills, and achieve and exercise independence. In other words, you are not merely teaching your child how to talk but also how to think, act, and be.

So without further ado, let's get on with chapter 1, "How to Recognize a Problem with Your Child's Speech, Language, or Communication Skills."

—Nicola

Chapter 1

# How to recognize a problem with your child's speech, language, or communication skills

**M**any parents have a gut feeling that there is something wrong with their child's speech, language, or communication development, but often it is difficult to know, first, whether or not you should be worried, and second, exactly where the problem lies.

Below are two checklists; the first is a brief age-related screening assessment (this, or something similar, might be used by the SLP at a child's initial assessment session) and the second is a list of behaviors and scenarios that should help you work out where your child's biggest communication challenges lie. Use the lists below to identify if there is an issue and what the priority area is, then you'll be able to navigate to a correlating section of the book for specific guidance.

## Checklist 1: Age-Related Screening Assessment

### A child of 12 months of age or less
A child of this age should see an SLP if they

- have difficulty with eating or drinking,
- are not responding to noises in the environment or your voice,
- are not looking at or interacting with familiar adults, and/or
- are not babbling at 12 months.

### A 2-year-old child
A child of this age should see an SLP if they

- cannot focus on an activity that they have chosen for more than a few seconds,
- cannot follow very simple instructions,
- cannot understand short phrases—for instance, "Get your coat" or "Where's teddy?,"
- are saying fewer than 50 words, and/or
- seem to have lost some of their skills.

### A 2½-year-old child
A child of this age should see an SLP if they

- have difficulty concentrating on an activity for more than a few seconds,
- cannot understand two key words in a sentence—for example, "Make the *baby sit*" or "Show me your *nose* and your *hair*," and/or
- are saying fewer than seventy-five words and not joining two words together.

(Note that at this age, speech sounds are still inconsistently spoken, and it is common for a child to find the following speech sounds tricky: "s," "sh," "f," "v," "ch," "j," "th" and "r.")

## A 3-year-old child

A child of this age should see an SLP if they

- are not able to concentrate on an activity led by an adult for a few seconds,
- have difficulty understanding three key words in a sentence—for example, "*Put teddy* under the *bed*,"
- are still only using single words and learned phrases, and/or
- are only understood by familiar adults.

## A 4-year-old child

A child of this age should see an SLP if they

- seem vacant when you talk to them or they repeat your sentence back,
- are not able to make a conversation and seem reluctant to communicate,
- seem to be still using only key words in a sentence and not using grammar, such as past and future tenses, and therefore sound like a younger child,
- do not understand or use concepts such as big/little or in/on/under,
- are not understood when they're talking, and/or
- aren't mixing with peers.

# Checklist 2: Which is my child's priority area?

## A child with attention and listening difficulties might[1]

- be easily distractible, unable to focus on an activity led by an adult, or even on something your child has chosen, for long enough to gain information from it,
- have difficulty sitting still,
- appear to rush around and find it hard to focus on one activity,
- be unable to assimilate two pieces of information at the same time—for instance, if your child is watching TV, they won't be able to listen to you calling their name and will seem as if they're ignoring you,

9

- be unable to complete a task,
- not recall information immediately after it has been given,
- daydream,
- not engage in group activities,
- need constant reminders from adults to look and listen, and/or
- be labeled as "disobedient" or "disruptive" because your child can't do what they are told.

## A child with difficulty understanding might

- repeat instructions rather than carry them out (known as echolalia),
- follow part of an instruction rather than the whole thing,
- appear not to listen when spoken to,
- appear quiet and withdrawn,
- show a lack of interest when stories are read,
- be labeled as "naughty" because they can't follow the instructions,
- answer questions incorrectly and inappropriately,
- wait for others to move before following an instruction when in a group,
- generally copy other children,
- rely on the use of gestures and other nonverbal clues,
- look slightly vacant when you talk to them,
- prefer to stick to an established routine and get upset or agitated when it changes, and/or
- be unable to understand complicated sentences and follow verbal instructions.

## A child who has difficulty talking might

- use a limited amount of words, relying on a reduced vocabulary,
- say only the key words in a sentence and miss the grammar,
- sound like a much younger child,
- repeat the same phrases over and over again,
- shorten long words and long sentences,

- frequently have trouble finding the right word and get stuck, or use a word that is closely related to the target word but not exact—for instance, using "house" for any building,
- be shy or withdrawn with other children or adults, especially if they perceive that they are expected to talk during an activity,
- use gestures, facial expressions, and body language to communicate,
- be very physical to get attention—for instance, by tapping or hitting other children,
- be frequently frustrated,
- be reluctant or refuse to answer direct questions, and/or
- have difficulty retelling a story or relaying information.

## A child with speech–sound problems might

- sound like a younger child,
- talk, but be difficult to understand,
- have difficulty making themselves understood to unfamiliar adults and look to their parents to interpret,
- use nonverbal communication (signs, gestures, facial expressions, pointing, and so on) to communicate,
- be frequently frustrated, and/or
- use the same word or sound over and over again.

## A child with social communication difficulties might

- appear to be a loner and spend a lot of time playing by themselves,
- have limited or inappropriate social communication (e.g., be quite physical rather than verbal, not respond when spoken to, pull an adult physically or put their hand on something they want),
- have inappropriate volume, speak in a monotone or talk too fast,
- talk about one subject for much of the time,
- not give eye contact during communication,
- be unable to play imaginatively with toys and instead do the same play routine over and over—for instance, lining up cars,

- not be able to take turns in a conversation,
- talk continuously, shout out, or find it difficult to take turns,
- make inappropriate comments that appear rude or obnoxious,
- be quiet or withdrawn but quite happy in their own little world,
- have difficulty sitting for group activities,
- not show things to adults or point, and/or
- prefer to follow a routine and may be anxious when the routine is abandoned.

## What to do if your child needs help

If you are concerned that your child may have a speech, language, or communication problem, get help early—the earlier the better. Talk to your pediatrician or local speech-language pathologist. This book doesn't replace the need to see a trained professional, but it gives you a head start in identifying your child's communication issues and enables you to begin to implement simple strategies that can help.

## What will a speech-language pathologist (SLP) do?

An SLP will see a child who has a difficulty in any of the areas listed below.

- Attention and listening
- Skills for understanding language and using expressive language
- Social communication skills
- Speech skills
- Voice problems
- Oral skills (problems with strength, range, and speed of oral movements)
- Eating and drinking issues
- Stuttering

The SLP will assess your child's skills to establish or confirm where the problem lies. We do this in many ways: through play, observation, standardized assessments, and discussion with key people. You will then be offered tailored advice, targets, and a program of exercises and training workshops designed to help achieve the targets. Your child's SLP will include the whole family as much as possible, and they will work together with other experts, such as teachers, pediatricians, occupational therapists, nursery caregivers, and so on, to provide an integrated service for your child.

## WHAT IS LANGUAGE AND HOW DOES IT DEVELOP?

Given how often I am grilled about first words, vocabulary, and general speech milestones by friends and family, it's clear to me that most parents want more information on how children develop speech, language, and communication skills. I always find that people are reassured if they feel informed, so here I will explain more fully what's going on in your baby's brain during the crucial first four years of life—while keeping things as simple as I can.

### What is language?

Speech, language, and communication involve a variety of skills.

- Attention and listening: how we focus and concentrate on the person talking in order to receive a message
- Comprehension: how we understand the language that we hear
- Expression: how we form words into sentences and use appropriate grammar to convey a message
- Speech/phonology: how we use sounds to make up a word
- Social skills and pragmatics: how we interact with someone to receive a message and use language appropriately to communicate, such as body language, eye contact, tone, volume, etc.
- Memory: how we remember and store words and sentences in our brain

The diagram below demonstrates this beautifully.

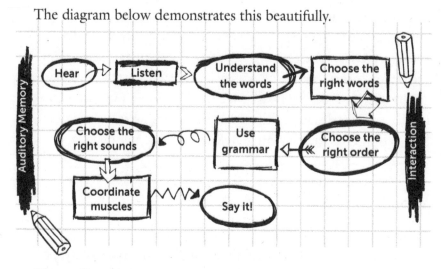

## How does language develop?

It's pretty amazing that children speak. It is thought to be the most complex skill human beings develop and we still don't understand it fully. Philosophers, psychologists, and linguists debate endlessly about what exactly enables a child to acquire language—is it nature or nurture? How is the brain wired in order to listen to and process language? Numerous models have been drawn to try to represent these processes, but I think the two diagrams below represent language development most clearly. The Language Cake shows the general outline of the components a child needs to acquire in order to speak, and the Language Tree shows this in more detail, along with what the parent can do to influence this process.

## The Language Cake

Imagine trying to serve a cake without a plate. It would crumble and disintegrate. In the illustration that follows, the plate represents the skills that need to be mastered before language can develop. These skills, the foundation for language, are showing an awareness of others, having a desire to communicate, listening, waiting, turn-taking, memory, attention, play (pretend play and imaginative/symbolic play), and eye contact. These preverbal skills are all essential to a greater or lesser degree, depending on the child, in order to acquire spoken language.

Once the skills shown on the plate are in place, children will start to respond to verbal language because they now have the tools to begin to understand spoken language. For instance, take the word *bye-bye*. Imagine a set of parents, frantically waving and saying, "Bye-bye, bye-bye" to their preverbal child. This child needs to have an awareness that someone is communicating with them, a desire to communicate back by looking, listening and attending/concentrating, remembering, taking a turn, etc., and then, when these skills are established, the child will begin to understand the word *bye-bye*, attempt to say it—possibly by saying "ba-ba" or "dye-dye" in the first instance—and then adjust it to "bye-bye" once their speech skills are developed.

I see a lot of children who aren't talking, and often their parents are desperate for me to start therapy that targets saying words. I have to explain to them that the preverbal skills shown on the Language Cake plate need to be addressed first. So, I might focus on playing turn-taking games or listening to environmental noises (e.g., the washing machine, the birds in the garden) to improve a child's attention and understanding. Only then can we proceed with actually saying words.

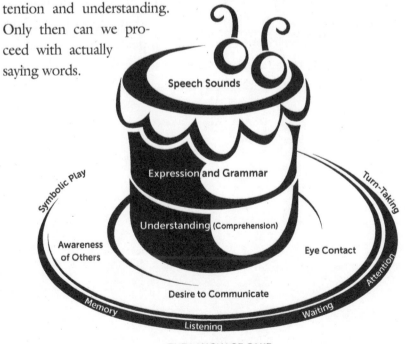

THE LANGUAGE CAKE

## The Language Tree

The Language Tree shows how the "Top Tips for Talking" (see page 17) directly influence a child's language development. The roots of the tree are attention/listening and understanding of language and thinking—without these, the tree would fall down. The tree then grows, and spoken language/expressive language appears. Words form the bulk of language—the tree trunk—and, from this, sentences emerge. The fruit and leaves on the tree are most noticeable to the eye and are what make it pretty—speech sounds and grammar are what make language sound pretty, but you could understand language without good speech sounds or eloquent grammar (in the same way you can grasp the meaning intended when a foreigner speaks broken English). Without sunshine, the tree would not grow at all. In this diagram, sunshine represents parental input and praise, and the rain represents the things a parent can do to help the tree to grow. In no particular order, these are create positive interactions; use single words and short sentences; allow time; give instructions in small steps; avoid lots of questions; offer choices; talk about the "here and now"; have realistic but high expectations; develop listening skills; repeat, repeat, repeat; be a Tuned-In Parent (see page 28); and use Say What You See (which you'll learn more about on pages 24–26).

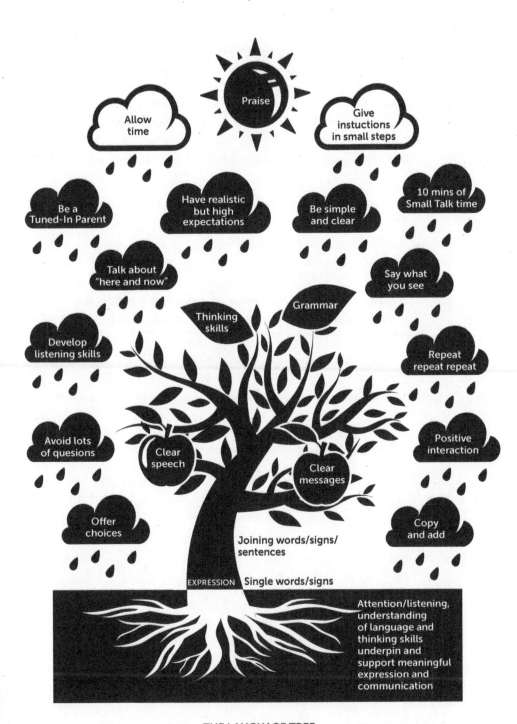

**THE LANGUAGE TREE**

## THE FIVE WAYS IN WHICH CHILDREN LEARN LANGUAGE

Research by British academics Judith Coupe O'Kane and Juliet Goldbart, who specialize in communication at Manchester Metropolitan University, concluded that there are five fundamental principles of how children learn language.[2]

- A child needs a reason to communicate.
- A child begins to use language when they understand that it's a better way to get what they want.
- A child learns language through meaningful interactions with an adult who is providing both appropriate models and appropriate content. This is NOT a passive process.
- A child needs an adult to provide repetition and clarification in order for them to develop the ability to decode what is being said.
- A child needs to develop cognitive and social skills alongside language skills in order to continue developing language.

## TOP TIPS FOR TALKING

Here are six of the best "Top Tips" you can start using right now to help a child with speech, language and communication delay.

Now that you can see how difficult learning to speak actually is, there are a few simple techniques that you can implement right away—even if you haven't yet had time to read the rest of the book. These skills will empower you to get the best out of your child and are relevant to every single interaction you have together, so aim to make them part of your daily routine.

And don't worry, I know that most parents never have a free moment, so these tips are super quick and effective. Ten minutes is all you need! I hope that if you find a small window you will just reach for this book and find these strategies for some speech-boosting inspiration.

## Top Tip for Talking 1

### Enjoy 10 minutes of Special Time every day

I tell parents to aim for a minimum of 10 minutes of dedicated one-on-one playtime with their child every day (this should be separate from reading a bedtime story together). It may sound shockingly short but it's achievable even for the busiest of parents and these 10 minutes of fun and games will make a big difference in your child's communication skills (and their emotional well-being, too). I want to emphasize that this is the bare minimum—if you have the luxury of spending three hours of uninterrupted quality time with your baby each day, while managing to maintain fun and enthusiasm, then do! This is an important point because it is quality, not quantity, that counts when it comes to Special Time.

Aiming for 10 minutes of uninterrupted time is crucial and achievable for most parents, and 10 minutes can easily turn into more when you are having fun!

### GETTING THE MOST OUT OF STORY TIME

A bedtime story should be additional to your 10 minutes of Special Time a day and should be done from a very early age—from birth, in fact. I find that many of the parents I meet at my clinic try to read to their babies every word of a book when, actually, for young babies, it's best to simply say one or two single words that relate to the pictures on the page. As you "tune in" to the level of your child's language and thought, you will be able to modify your storytelling accordingly—first reading one word or line from each page, then the whole story.

Don't forget to point out parts of the images your child might be interested in that may not always relate to the text—a picture of a dog or tractor, perhaps. Use your baby's finger to point to these things, as it encourages your child to look at the same thing you are looking at and talking about.

Seek out books with a catchphrase repeated on every page—for example, *Brown Bear, Brown Bear, What Do You See?* by Bill Martin Jr. and Eric Carle or, for older children, *We're Going on a Bear Hunt* by Michael Rosen and Helen Oxenbury. Or if you have a favorite book that doesn't have a repetitive line in it, simply add one yourself. I love the book *Where's Spot?* by Eric Hill, and tell parents to say, "Where's Spot?" each time they turn the page, even though, amazingly, it's not in the text. The goal is that your children should know the catchphrase so well that you can pause as you turn the page, and they will say the punch line for you, learning new words and grammar as they go.

Lastly, photo albums can work just as well as storybooks. Initially, simply name the people in the pictures, then add more detail. For example, first you might say "Mummy," then this might become "Mummy swimming" and finally "Mummy swimming in the ocean on vacation last summer" (see page 266, "How to Choose and Get the Best Out of Your Storybooks," for more hints and tips on reading stories).

## Top Tip for Talking 2

### When your child plays, remove screens

This piece of advice is very important, and more difficult to achieve than you would imagine. It centers on your child's not being distracted by screens while playing. We all know how easy it is to be distracted when we try to sit down and focus on one particular task, and for children, more often than not, it is a screen that they're distracted by. And, inevitably, they end up focusing on the screen instead of their play or your model for language.

Remember this Top Tip during your Special Time, too; you are busy and it's not my aim to make you feel guilty, but I'd encourage you to try to figure out when in your day the windows of opportunity arise and make the most of them. It could be between supper and the start of the bedtime routine, or the 10 minutes before you unload the dishwasher. Try to constantly remind yourself that your Special Time has to be quality time.

Research tells us that many of us parents are prioritizing chores over uninterrupted one-on-one time with our children. I know that life can be terribly busy, but try not to multitask or get distracted during your Special Time. Think about a recent time you spent with your little one; did you have your phone in your hand, the TV on, or Twitter at your side while you played or talked? I often have to remind my husband to put his phone down when he plays with our daughter, Jess, as it seems to have been surgically stitched to his hand!

I must admit I'm guilty of multitasking, too. Only the other evening, I was reading Jess a bedtime story while watching television at the same time. It was so natural, sitting in the living room with the TV on, that it was a few minutes before I realized I was shortchanging Jess and turned it off.

Ensure the TV is switched off and phones are out of reach and on silent. When there is background noise, the words you say become indistinct and it's difficult for your child to focus on you—and, don't forget, you are your child's best role model for language. All ears should be on you, so they only have one source of information to process.

Sit down with your child, and be sure you are at the same eye level and face-to-face. If your child is little, sit them in a baby bouncer or prop baby up with pillows on the bed while you sit opposite, otherwise just sit on the floor together. Either way, it is important that young babies are well supported—you'll get more out of your child if they don't have to focus on balancing in order to achieve head control, or on sitting or standing while trying to concentrate on you.

## Top Tip for Talking 3

### Keep your language simple and clear

SLPs agree that understanding language is the key to good language development. The more your child understands, the better their language will be and the more they will want to say. Once your baby can understand that something that is fluffy and says "woof, woof" is a *dog*, they can then begin to say the word. So, we must use our words clearly as a model for our babies. For example, "Look, a cat. Meow, meow, cat." (Read more on modeling words on page 82.)

Parents often fail to appreciate just how *new* everything is to their babies. We as adults have been chitchatting for years and years—I, for one, love to chat—but imagine how that must sound to a baby. You are essentially bombarding them with strange, unknown sounds that, to them, have absolutely no meaning. This must be even more confusing than if, say, you were abroad listening to people talk in a language you had never heard before, because at least you'd be able to understand the body language, facial expressions, and social context.

The best way to help your little one start to make sense of the world is by feeding them bite-size morsels of language at the right level. So, when your little one is under the age of one, for example, try to communicate in a very simple way using a lot of repetition.

Focus on the key words in a sentence and don't worry too much about using correct grammar. A sentence like "The teddy has fallen out of the stroller" should be simplified to "Teddy fall down," depending on the level of the child's language.

Many parents might worry about adapting the grammar of a sentence, but as your child's language grows, your own language naturally expands and becomes more grammatically advanced alongside your child's. Talking in this simplified way will help your little one begin to understand what these entirely new words and sounds mean.

## CASE STUDY: LINKING WORD AND ACTION

Owen has been taking his son, Laurie, swimming every week since he was eight weeks old. Right from the start Owen learned to say a set phrase to Laurie whenever he dunked him in the water. Several weeks into the course, Owen noticed that Laurie recognized the phrase "Laurie, ready, go!" and knew it meant he was about to get wet. Even if Owen said these words on dry land, like in the living room, Laurie would blink his eyes and hold his breath in preparation for the water. This proves just how quickly a child can link words and actions together, demonstrating beautifully how a baby of just three months old begins to grasp our language.

## Top Tip for Talking 4

### Repeat, repeat, repeat

Do you remember your school teacher drilling into you rules such as "*I* before *E* except after *C*" or, later on, Spanish phrases such as "¿Cómo te llamas?" If you do, this is because repeating words and ideas over and over again helps them to stick in your mind. So, applying this rule to language development, we have to say things, repeat them, and stress the words we want the child to learn.

In fact, children love to hear information being repeated (for example, when you tell the same story for the hundredth time or sing repeatedly about five little ducks who went swimming one day, over the hills and far away . . .). This may be tedious for you but it is a highly effective way for your little one to begin to understand the language that you are teaching them.

However, it is important to try to be consistent with the words or phrases that your child hears. For example, there are hundreds of ways to say that something is "small"—such as "little," "tiny," "itty-bitty," and so on—but your child will learn quicker if you drill into them just one such word, so try to pick one and stick to it in the early stages of language development. They will pick up the others later, don't worry.

## USING WORDS IN CONTEXT

A study I once read suggested that a child would need to hear a word being spoken in its context at least 500 times before they will understand what the word means, and many more times again before they will begin to attempt to say it. I once told a parent this and she, quite understandably, asked if this meant she could simply say "cup" 500 times in a row and her baby would suddenly be able to say it. An interesting idea! The answer is no, but do try to repeat certain words often and, most importantly, in context. For example, say "up" each time you pick up your baby, repeat "down, down, down" when you go down the stairs, "open the door" when you're getting into the car or "shake, shake, shake" for a rattle. Doing this each time will help your baby learn the word and also reinforce the context in which that word is meaningfully used.

## Top Tip for Talking 5

### Stay one step ahead

As your child gets older and progresses through the phases of language and speech development, as a parent you need to stay one step ahead. So, ideally, you would be able to identify which phase of communication your child is in and know what is coming next—then you can continuously encourage your little one to move forward to the next phase. This book will help you to do that. Being aware of where you're headed will help enormously!

## Top Tip for Talking 6

### Say What You See

If you only take one thing away from this book, it should be this: Say What You See. This is THE most important technique you can use with your child. I drone on and on about Say What You See because parents need to master this technique in order to promote their child's language development. Simply put, the idea is that language develops through play. So, watch your child play, think about what they might be thinking, and provide a comment to put *their thoughts* into words. This might *sound* easy, but it can actually be quite tricky and it takes a lot of practice to get good at it. Using the Say What You See technique helps children feel relaxed and secure, exposes them to language relevant to their play, and enables them to receive positive responses as they attempt to communicate.

All you do is give a gentle running commentary of what your child is doing and what is happening at that moment in time. It involves following your child's lead, observing them closely to see what they are interested in, and commenting and then pausing to give space for your child to respond. We can often talk too much or ask too many questions without giving our children a chance to speak. So, rather than saying, "What are you doing?," "Did Dolly fall down?," you should say, "Dolly's drinking her milk. Whoops! She fell off the chair. Poor Dolly. Ah, May's cuddling the dolly." (Incidentally, I always use the child's name—in this case, "May"— or I omit the name, saying, for instance, "cuddle the dolly," rather than use pronouns such as "you" or "I," which, in this case, would be "You're cuddling the dolly." To use these latter pronouns can be confusing for the child. For advice on when to use "I" and "you," see Pronouns, page 174).

This powerful technique helps your child to focus on their activity for longer (and the longer they stay with an activity, the more they will learn), become involved in what they're doing, and link what they hear to what they are doing or thinking. Crucially, it also helps children feel confident and relaxed because it avoids putting pressure on them to talk or give answers, and you will find that they are more likely to babble or talk in response to your comments when they feel under no obligation to speak.

Having said all that, it's not nearly as easy to hold back as it sounds. We naturally want to test, question, and direct our children. For example, if a child were to bang blocks together, perhaps not playing with them in the traditional way, instinctively you would want to say, "Build me a tower," but what you should say is, "Bang, bang, bang go the bricks." By saying "bang, bang, bang" you are verbalizing your child's thoughts, showing them your interest and valuing what they're doing rather than directing their play—so you become a great playmate rather than a teacher. And next time they repeat the action or play sequence, they will hear your voice in their head, almost like a scratched record, and eventually want to say it for themselves.

These Top Tips require you to learn a lot of new information and you are unlikely to take it all in at once. Please don't worry. You're learning as your child learns—in bite-size pieces! Try to incorporate one of these techniques at a time into your daily routine until they become second nature. Practice makes perfect!

## SAY WHAT YOU SEE WORKS FOR ALL AGES

A work colleague of mine tells a wonderful story about her grandson, who is nine. She took him to the park and he said, "Granny, will you do that thing where you say what I am doing?" And she remembered having continuously used Say What You See when he was a child. She willingly obliged, saying, "Up, up, up the steps. Sitting down at the top of the slide. Getting ready . . . wheeeee, down you go." He was clearly loving the fact that she was totally involved and enjoying his play, which gave him a sense of confidence and security.

This just proves that Say What You See is for children of all ages and, honestly, all children love it. Sometimes when you carry out this technique with a child for the first time, they look at you in amazement and then do something else to see what you'll say. Obviously, if they were to throw the toy you'd discipline as usual, but that's the beauty of this technique: You can dip in and out of it as much as you like throughout your day. Please, please, try it today!

# WHAT TYPE OF PARENT ARE YOU?

I know that you're reading this book to learn all about your child's communication, but the last word in this chapter is actually all about you! Throughout this book you will find lots more games and activities (under the heading "Top Tip for Talking") to help your child learn these skills. And as you, the parent, are fundamental to helping your child become a great communicator, let's now look at your own parenting style and how to adjust it to benefit your child. Get ready to be brutally honest with yourself—if you're not sure, ask your partner or a trusted friend what kind of parent they think you are!

In the textbook *It Takes Two to Talk* by Jan Pepper and Elaine Weitzman, one of the most useful chapters confronts the sensitive issue of the parents' communication style and how it can impact their child's speech, language and communication development. The authors describe seven types of parent and explain that, throughout the day, a parent may dip in and out of all seven "types" but usually has one dominant parenting style. Read the descriptions below, which have been adapted from Pepper and Weitzman's book,[3] and see if you can spot yourself.

## The Director

The role of director has the parent leading and controlling a child's daily interactions. The parent does most of the talking and tells the child what to do and how to do it. For example, Robert wants to find the page with the monster in his favorite book but his dad is playing the director role, insisting that they read the book page by page.

## The Tester

In this role, the parent asks a lot of questions in order to see what the child has learned. But constant testing doesn't help the child learn—a child learns best when they're having fun and their parents are tuned in to their interests.

### The Entertainer

When in this role, the parent tends to take the lead, doing most of the talking *and* playing, and leaving little opportunity for the child to interact and be part of the fun. However, children need to be actively involved to learn.

### The Helper

The Helper does everything for the child, from finishing their sentences to answering questions on their behalf. But when parents are too quick to help, they may not find out how much the child can communicate and what really interests them.

### The Mover

This role may be adopted by a busy parent who has 101 things to do that take priority over communicating with the child. This parent often does not notice when the child is trying to show or tell them something.

### The Watcher

Sometimes, parents would like to interact with the child but aren't sure how to join in, so end up watching or commenting from a distance. But to learn language, children need to interact with their parents.

### The Tuned-In Parent

This parent is tuned in to the child's interests, needs and abilities. A Tuned-In Parent gives children opportunities to start an interaction and then responds immediately, with interest.

Out of these seven types, the Tuned-In Parent is the one to aspire to. You can't be a Tuned-In Parent all the time, but try to play this role more often—be honest and ask yourself if you talk too much, fool around too much, continuously test your child, or help your child too often.

You are your child's most valuable resource when it comes to learning to communicate, so please do try to tune in to being a Tuned-In Parent.

# Chapter 2

# What to do when . . . your baby isn't communicating with you

You're sitting at playgroup and all the other 6-month-old babies in your peer group are gazing adoringly at their mothers, seemingly fascinated by what their friends are doing and are making all manner of wonderful *ooe*, *eee*, and *ah* noises with a raspberry thrown in for good measure. Your baby, meanwhile, isn't saying a peep. This isn't a one-off occurrence. You might have noticed it over a period of weeks in different settings, leaving you wondering why your baby isn't babbling when everyone else's is.

Let's go back to the start. Many adults might think that the time before a baby's words emerge is irrelevant; that the sounds a baby makes are chaotic, arbitrary, and meaningless. This is far from the truth. Between the ages of 0 to 18 months, our tiny tots are forming the building blocks they need to be able to use words and language. In other words, the pre-babble or preverbal phase of moaning, groaning, screeching, squealing, staring into your eyes, and squawking for attention is absolutely essential and, as a Tuned-In Parent, you can identify and reward your baby's attempts to communicate, helping them on their journey toward spoken words.

Interestingly, this journey starts far earlier than you might think: At 24 weeks in utero, your baby's ear is now structurally complete, and researchers believe that even at 16 weeks' gestation, these tiny tots can hear sounds from outside the womb.

Neurotypical babies are born instinctively sociable and can interact with you from the day they're born by copying you—if you stick out your tongue, so will they, and when they are crying, they are telling you that they are either in pain or discomfort (due to a dirty nappy, feeling too hot or too cold, and so on), or feeling tired or hungry. Crying noises are made of vowel sounds such as "ah," "ooo," and "uh." And, before long, your baby will start to use these vowel sounds and experimental noises as a way to "talk" and here begins pre-babble, a way of communicating that must be responded to in order for the babble phase to start.

So, let's think about how your baby is interacting. This will tune you into what they are or aren't doing. Early on, their only method of communication is to gaze into their parent's eyes or to cry.

There are four types of cry, each meaning something different. Can you detect these types of cry in your young child?

## THE LISTEN, WAIT, RESPOND TECHNIQUE

Have you ever really listened to your baby cry? Usually, we're so quick to jump up in a panic and cuddle them that we often forget to actually listen. Next time your baby cries, listen hard for just ten to thirty seconds to the type of cry they are making so that you will gradually feel more confident in interpreting their cries and figuring out what they want. The only cry that must be addressed immediately is the pain cry, which is very distinct so you can't mistake it for something else—there will be no doubt that your baby is in pain.

### Types of cry

The types of cries your baby makes are

- pain cry: a sharp scream followed by a moment of no breathing, and another sharp scream,
- discomfort cry: a whiny sound, almost like a fake cry, which doesn't stop when the baby is picked up,
- hunger cry: a low-pitched cry that rises and falls with a rhythm. It usually gets progressively louder and the baby can't be calmed down. The baby might root for the breast or suck on their hand at the same time, and
- tired cry: a soft, rhythmic, moaning cry as the baby tries to settle to go to sleep.

Over time, these cries turn into spoken noises or simple vowel sounds. Cue the next communication phase!

## ARE CRIES BEGINNING TO SOUND LIKE VOWEL SOUNDS?

It may surprise you to learn that newborn babies are virtually silent—unless they are crying—because they haven't yet learned how to make any other sounds. Crying noises are made of vowel sounds—"ah," "hoo," "ooo," "uh." And, before long, your baby will start to use these vowel sounds as a way to "talk," so you will begin to hear little "aahs" and "uurs" popping out as they kick on the play mat. (This could happen at about 10 to 12 weeks).

I bet you didn't think that crying is nature's way of enabling a baby to climb the language development ladder! Crying is the first spoken means of communication, and even though there are no fully formed words within a baby's cries, the seeds of those words are there and are encouraged to grow through the crying process.

But there are also ways that you can help to nurture these seeds. The best way is by playing games, and below are a few suggestions.

**Top Tip Time** **Encouraging early vowel sounds**

We have already established that crying noises sound like more desperate vowels, so the next step is to play games involving vowel noises anytime from around 3 months onward. Try the following games.

- Every time you hug your baby say, "Ahhh." My daughter at age 2½ was still saying, "Ahhh" when we cuddled.
- Fall to the floor and say, "Argh!" Children are highly motivated by sound and movement, so can you imagine how rewarding it would be to a baby to see a grown adult fall to the floor, saying, "Argh!" right in front of their face?
- Prop your baby up so they can see you clearly, then spin around and say, "Eeee."
- Yawn in a very exaggerated way, saying "Hurrrh" with a big stretch. You could stretch your baby's arms up at the same time.
- Sit your baby on your lap, facing you. Bounce them up and say, "Weeeee" and then lower them down, saying, "Oooooohhhh."
- Continue to use "motherese" (see page 43) when you're face-to-face with your little one. Talk to your baby about anything and everything: "We're going to see Maisie and Carrie today at the café." Then wait for your baby to say something. Then respond again, "Yes, you're right. We'll have to wrap up warm—it's cold outside."

The key with these games is to play them a few times to establish the routine and to get your baby familiar with the noise that is paired with the action. Then, play the game again and pause before your big finale, enabling your baby to join in and attempt appropriate sounds, too—which may take some time. Once your child realizes that their sounds are intentional and meaningful (so that, if they say, "Eee," they are rewarded by your spinning around in response to them), they will continue to move forward with their communication. This is another anticipation game, where you are anticipating your baby's movement or noise as they interact with you during the game. It can be noisy, but great fun!

## CAN YOU HEAR YOUR BABY MAKING LOTS OF DIFFERENT VOWEL SOUNDS?

There are five vowel letters in the English alphabet (*A, E, I, O, U*). But in the speech and language therapy world there are many more vowel sounds—depending on the accent, it's somewhere between eleven and twenty. Say the following four words and listen to how different the letter "a" sounds each time: *father, cat, about, pay.*

So, when you hear your baby begin to experiment with sounds and noises, trying to "talk," it is a wide range of vowel sounds that you will hear—"ah," "ur," "ooo," "ei," "uh," "aya," and so on, rather than *A, E, I, O,* and *U.* As I previously mentioned, vowel sounds are derived from crying noises. I suppose the best way to explain this is that they are like spoken crying noises that the baby uses to experiment with finding their voice.

Once your baby starts to use them, it's really important that you react and reward them by smiling, talking back and looking at your child to engage them and show them that you are listening. Say things like, "Are you telling me a story?" and "And then what happened?" This way, you are encouraging your baby to say more.

## HOW BABIES BEGIN TO LEARN WORDS

The other day, a friend of mine said, "Guess what? Milly [6 months] has started saying "iya" [as in "Hi-ya"]. Can it really be true?" Well, the answer is yes! Initially, a child says something by accident, which sounds like a real word. At 6 months, it was probably the case that Milly was saying this word accidentally, as part of her experimental speech, but because her parent was so delighted, Milly was rewarded by having the word said back to her—for example, "Iya, iya, Milly." Then, sooner or later, Milly would have begun to understand that she was communicating with her parent and repeated the word—randomly initially, then she began to use it in the correct context. The realization that you and your baby are intentionally communicating with each other is really exciting.

**Top Tip Time** **More vowels, please!**

Try the following games to encourage your baby to say some vowel sounds.

- Get down on the floor so that you're at your baby's level and play with a toy you know they really like, preferably something that makes a noise. You could even lie on the floor together and encourage a bit of tummy time. Don't make a sound yourself but create a sound from the toy. Don't give your baby eye contact unless you sense that they are not looking at you or the toy and, if this is the case, move into their line of vision again until they look at you. The idea is to encourage them to get your attention by using their voice. If they make a sound, respond immediately by bringing the toy closer to them and showing it to them. Give them a big kiss and the toy to play with and say, "You're so clever; you were calling Mummy." If your baby doesn't make a sound, respond to a physical movement—for example, a wave of their arms or an excited kick. Keep rewarding their efforts and respond extra enthusiastically when they do make a sound.

- Make various vowel sounds to your baby in the mirror and wait to see if they copy you. In the first instance, you could try "ooo," "eee," and "ah." Say the sounds your baby makes back, too.

- Sing songs that include vowel sounds to your baby—this will not only help to develop the vowel sounds in their vocabulary but also boost their listening skills. A favorite with my patients is the classic "Old MacDonald Had a Farm," simply because of the chorus, "E-I-E-I-O," which is made entirely of vowel sounds. The key is to sing it very slowly so your baby can listen and join in. Another good song is "Row, Row, Row Your Boat," with the version of the ending that goes "If you see a crocodile, don't forget to scream—argh!"

- It sounds obvious, but you can say, "Aah" whenever you cuddle your baby or a teddy, and say, "Ooo" whenever you see anything surprising or interesting.

- If you're really motivated, you could make simple and bold flash cards for your baby. Try a ghost for "ooo," a mouse for "eee," and a crocodile for "argh."

It might be that your child, for some reason, doesn't seem interested in looking at or interacting with you. Although eye contact per se isn't the be-all and end-all of excellent communication skills—and some people who have poor eye contact can still communicate extremely well—a child who engages with others and learns to listen to people who are talking to them has a huge advantage when it comes to developing social skills, learning to talk and learning in general.

## IS YOUR BABY INTERACTING AND MAKING EYE CONTACT WITH YOU?

From the moment your baby is born, they instinctively want to look at your face, in fact baby's brains are preprogrammed to be attracted to looking at people's faces. Can you imagine hearing the same voice for nine months and not knowing where the sound is coming from? Sure enough, soon after birth, your baby will begin to actively check out the source of the sound—your face. Amazingly, within 15 hours of birth, a baby can recognize which face their mother's voice is coming from. At birth, a baby is able to focus at a distance of 8 to 12 inches (20–30 cm), which is the rough distance between a baby's face and their parent's when they are feeding—perfect planning by Mother Nature.

Establishing good eye contact with your baby helps you develop a strong social and emotional bond, encourages your baby to look at your face to see where the sound comes from and, a few weeks down the line, copy and experiment with their own voice.

## HOW EYE CONTACT DEVELOPS

Outlined below is the developmental pattern for eye contact.

- A newborn is able to look for short periods at a human face and is attracted by movement.
- At 2 months, a baby will "lock" on to a human face, especially when the face is accompanied by a voice, and can use their eyes to track between two people, objects, or patterns—even at some distance.
- At 4 to 6 months, a baby recognizes familiar people by smiling at them, but is also drawn toward the novelty of a new face or object.

## Why is eye contact important for early communication?

I am reminded of the importance of eye contact every time I take case histories from parents who have children with speech and language problems. I notice that when I break eye contact, the person stops speaking. When I maintain eye contact, the person continues talking, knowing that I am interested in what they have to say.

The same idea relates to children. When a baby gives and receives good eye contact, they begin to gather information about language through watching your facial expression, gestures, and signs. This is the beginning of social interaction.

## Reduced eye contact

This is a characteristic that is often associated with children who have autism. It is, of course, one of very many characteristics associated with autism. First, please don't assume if your child isn't looking at you that they have autism, because conversely many children who give eye contact can still be diagnosed with autism. (For more information about autism and a checklist of signs to watch out for, see pages 277–79.)

In most cases, a baby or child not giving eye contact is simply another phase in the developmental process and no cause for concern. During my years of working with children, I've noticed that while babies tend to gaze adoringly at their parents for the first two months, at about 8 to 10 weeks a baby's eyesight improves and they start actively looking into the wider environment and becoming fascinated with what's going on around them—rather than with you! Your baby's interest in faces will return as quickly as it went and, after a few weeks, they'll be desperate to look at people again and start flirting and crowd-pleasing with beautiful wide eyes and beaming smiles all over again.

### TUNED IN TO HUMAN CONTACT

Babies as young as 3 months can tell the difference between a happy voice and a sad voice. At this age they can also tell human voices from other sounds. A research team from the Institute of Psychiatry at King's College, London, studying babies from 3 to 7 months, found that coughing, sneezing, yawning, lapping water (reminiscent of bath time), and the squeaking of toys all activated a part of the brain known to process speech.[1] But human sounds lit it up far more.

**Top Tip Time** **Encouraging your baby to look at you**

One of the most amazing things that a baby can do at birth is to copy oral movements that their parent makes. For example, if the parent pokes out their tongue or makes an "ooo" shape with their mouth, the baby will, too. Give it a try! Also try the Top Tip games below with babies that are 3 to 4 months and older. Actively encourage your baby to look at you and engage with you when you play these games.

- Wear funny glasses, hats, noses, wigs, or bright lipstick. (Go on, dads—don't be shy!)
- Look in the mirror and make funny faces at each other. Wait for your baby to try to copy you.
- Sing some songs and rhymes in the mirror and point to the appropriate body parts. Here's a rhyme to try.

   *Two little eyes to look around,*
   *Two little ears to hear each sound,*
   *One little nose to smell what's sweet,*
   *One little mouth that tastes what to eat.*

- Below is a song that's great for this activity.

   *I look in the mirror and who do I see?*
   *Who is that baby, looking at me?*
   *I look in the mirror and who do I see?*
   *That face in the mirror is me.*

- Pick up a noisy or sparkly toy and move it slowly from left to right in front of your baby's face. Go slowly, so that you can see their eyes tracking the toy. Make it disappear behind your head or back and wait for your baby to make eye contact. Give them a big smile and say, "Yes, you are looking at Mummy!"
- Play peekaboo. Initially, use a gauzy, transparent scarf or piece of fabric (muslins are great for this) and briefly trail it over your face, so your baby can see your face and then you

momentarily disappear. As your face is covered, start saying "Peek-aaaa . . ." then pop out and say, "boo!" Babies often find this hilarious and will give lots of smiles. You can then try trailing the fabric over baby's face and use the same routine—encourage your baby to pull it off. Once they get the hang of it you can make the game more interactive by leaving a long pause after saying, "Peek-a- . . . (pause)" for your baby to make an excited movement or a noise (and then you say, "boo")—the baby's noise should eventually become a "boo." This type of game is known as an anticipation game—you are anticipating that your baby will say a sound or attempt a word at a particular point.

- Try sticking a sticker next to your eyes or on your nose to encourage your baby to look at you—a simple, cheap, and effective idea.

## PARENT-FACING STROLLERS

Wondering whether to buy a forward-facing or parent-facing (also known as rear-facing) stroller for your baby? I would always recommend a parent-facing one, as studies have shown that parents are twice as likely to talk to their children when they are facing them, which could have a big impact on language development.

This was definitely true in my case. I had the use of two strollers, one of which was parent-facing, the other forward-facing. When my daughter Jess sat in the parent-facing stroller, I noticed that I talked to her a lot more (perhaps too much!). I'd basically think aloud, saying things like "I wonder if Daddy's home?," "Mmm, what shall we have for lunch?," or "Oh, I think there's some yummy cheese in the fridge." However, when Jess was forward-facing, I'd have the same thoughts but not bother to say them out loud.

And I'm not alone in this. Research carried out by Dr. Suzanne Zeedyk, developmental psychologist at the University of Dundee, examined interactions between parents and their infants who were seated in both parent-facing and forward-facing strollers.[2] The report concluded that parents are twice as likely to talk to children in parent-facing strollers, which could have an impact on language development. I recommend a parent-facing stroller if at all possible.

## What if . . . your baby is terrified of strangers?

At 6 to 8 months your baby will go through a very social phase but, confusingly, this will almost definitely be followed by a phase of clinginess and stranger anxiety. Babies start to only have eyes for the people they know well, usually their mothers or fathers, and experts suggest that this is a basic survival instinct that maintains the powerful bond between the child and the person who feeds, clothes, and comforts them and keeps them safe. All babies will experience this, whether it's for one day, one week, or several months. Thankfully, there are a few things you can do to help your baby through this tricky time.

**Top Tip Time** **Stranger anxiety**

During this period, try to expose your baby to as many people as possible, in as many different places as possible. Go to baby groups, family gatherings, and friends' houses. Encourage your little one to be held by others—only if they want to—and interact with them. Your hard work will pay off when you don't have a child stuck to your hip for months on end!

## HELPING YOUR LITTLE ONE FOCUS

Remember that if your little one can't sit up yet, while sitting on your lap and working hard to hold their head up, they won't be able to focus well on the words and sounds you say because all their energy will be going into their balance. In this instance, lay them down on their back so that their body is well supported. They are likely to listen to many more sounds and noises this way.

## HAVE YOU HAD A CHAT?

If you've been practicing the exercises given in this book so far, your little one will now understand that they are making sounds that people are interested in because they are being rewarded with smiles and replies from you for their attempts to talk. At this stage, you will notice a boom in the amount of vocalizations your child makes as they intentionally attempt to "talk"—this is a very important step.

So how do you create a conversation? It's all about the art of turn-taking, and here's how to do it.

**Top Tip Time** **Turn-taking—encouraging a babble chat!**

Have a chat with your baby—yes, I know it seems far-fetched but you really can do this before they can talk, and if your child is struggling with their speech, language, and communication skills, try doing this as much as you possibly can!

Wait for your child to say something. Once they have finished "talking," leave a slight pause in case there is more. Then make a comment yourself, such as "Yes, it really is cold today." Try to keep your utterance at a similar length to that of your baby's, or slightly shorter, and wait for your tiny talker to say some more. If they cut you off, let them. Hopefully, you will now be turn-taking in a bit of "small talk." Try to keep this "conversation" going for as long as possible, as many as 5 to 10 exchanges, by giving lots of smiles and eye contact to show that you are finding their story incredibly interesting. You are being a Tuned-In Parent. Bravo.

As your little chats develop, you might hear vowel sounds, or screams, or even some consonant sounds, but the key to having a conversation is looking at them, listening and waiting. If your baby doesn't say anything, say something yourself, then simply wait. So, you might start with "Where's Rhodri gone?" Wait . . . "Where is he?" Wait . . . Wait again . . . "We took him to school." Wait . . . "Ah," says the baby and you immediately respond: "Yes, he's at school." Then wait some more. If a sound is made, either copy it or use some "motherese" to try to expand it.

Work on turn-taking when you are alone with your child and when there is no background noise—it's much harder to get your little one to "share" the conversation when brothers and sisters are running around! A good time to practice is when you are in proximity, such as during nappy changing, mealtimes, or bath time.

## Play Copycat

A very important part of developing a conversation is encouraging your child to copy the sounds they hear from you, another family member, or another child. Copying is an important skill to learn. If we can't copy others, how can we learn to speak? Copying also involves cooperation and interaction between two people—an essential part of communication. We usually teach a child to copy nonverbally before we encourage them to copy verbally.

I am a big believer in the value of playdates, as they give your little one the opportunity to spend time with other children, whether they are younger, older, or the same age. Did you ever notice your baby reaching out to touch the other children and then beginning to copy their noises and actions? Whether it's a cough or a scream or just a gesture, this copycat play is an important part of learning to speak.

# MOTHERESE

When we talk to infants, regardless of the language we speak, most adults alter their voices to attract the infant's attention, use short, simple sentences coupled with higher pitch and exaggerated intonation, and talk at a much slower rate to communicate effectively. This is usually known as "motherese" or baby talk or, in the scientific community, as infant-directed or child-directed speech. Research tells us that babies are pre-programmed to listen to such coochie-coo voices and, as parents, we often naturally and unconsciously talk to our babies like this to help them tune in to our speech. It's Mother Nature's way of encouraging that parent–baby bond.

When we use motherese we speak in short, slow sentences with repetitive words, we stretch out vowel sounds, add vowel sounds (e.g., doggy) and exaggerate intonation patterns, making our singsong speech more attractive to a baby's ear than a flat voice. (Don't worry if you end up saying "doggy" or "horsey" for some time. Some people disapprove of teaching children these "childish" words, but it does no harm and, before long, your little one will start correcting you, which is when you'll know it's time to use the proper word.)

When you are chatting to your baby using motherese, you shouldn't worry too much about the length of your sentences. However, when you want to help your baby learn something new, stop, say it clearly, and simply and repeat it. The following is an example of how to use motherese and teach new words at the same time: "Let's go into the kitchen and see what's in the fridge for lunch. What about a nice ham sandwich?" Then, when you get out the bread and show it to your baby, instead of saying, "Here's the bread," stop, say it clearly and simply and repeat it: "Bread, it's bread. Bread on the plate." By pausing, simplifying, and repeating the single word "bread" you are adapting your motherese and teaching a new word. You may think your tiny baby is too young to learn new words, but I can guarantee that you are doing this subconsciously already. You may be talking to your baby about their other parent at certain points throughout the day, saying things like "I wonder what Mummy/Daddy's doing? They might be getting in the car and driving home" (motherese). When the other parent actually comes in and picks up your baby, say, "Daddy. Daddy's home" or "Mummy. Mummy's home" (adapted motherese). This teaches your baby a potential first word—"Mummy" or "Daddy."

## Why "motherese" boosts speech

Researchers have long known that babies prefer to be spoken to in a singsong manner associated with motherese. But Erik Thiessen of Carnegie Mellon University has revealed that infant-directed speech also helps infants *learn words more quickly* than normal adult speech.[3]

In a series of experiments, he and his colleagues exposed 8-month-old infants to fluent speech made up of nonsense words. The researchers assessed whether, after listening to the fluent speech for less than 2 minutes, infants had been able to learn the words. The infants who were exposed to fluent speech with the exaggerated intonation contour characteristic of infant-directed speech, or motherese, learned to identify the words more quickly than infants who heard fluent speech spoken in a more monotone fashion.

## ENCOURAGING THE BUILDING BLOCKS FOR SPEECH

I remember once I was in a swimming pool changing room with Jess and another mum who had a 6-year-old boy with severe autism. As I tried to wrestle Jess into her swimsuit, as usual, she started to fuss and moan, and this little lad on the other side of the room began to copy her. I said to his mum, "Oh wow, he's copying my little girl's noises," and she hadn't really clocked that he was doing this. He was 6 and hadn't spoken a meaningful word yet. This was the first intentional noise his mother had ever heard him make and she was delighted. This was the stage of communication he was at—copying vowel sounds. I found it fascinating because it reaffirmed to me that children need to go through these crucial building blocks before they use real words.

## IS YOUR BABY MAKING EXPERIMENTAL NOISES?

Once your baby has acquired a range of vowel sounds and is becoming confident and competent at using them, the noises you hear them make will become more adventurous and amusing (this could happen at around 3 to 4 months). They are beginning to experiment with their lips, tongue, and jaw in order to make many different sounds, such as screams and squeals, blowing raspberries, grunts, and growls and you may hear some consonant sounds appearing (all sounds that are not vowels—more about these in the next chapter). They will also be experimenting with volume and tone—here's where the tuneful nature of your coochie-coo voice begins to pay off, as you'll hear your baby beginning to imitate your intonation patterns.

My daughter growled a lot. Even my friend's 2-year-old noticed and one day said, "She thinks she's a lion!" I had to consider why she was making this noise as, I can assure you, it wasn't a noise she was copying from my husband or me. My explanation was that the growls make a lovely vibration in the throat and therefore gave Jess a lot of tactile feedback—so she wanted to say "grrr" again and again! Such noises are experimental and therefore they don't have to be a proper English sound.

The purpose of these experimental sounds is to prepare the mouth for consonant sounds by building the neurological pathways from the brain to the jaw, lips, and tongue (known as the articulators). In other words, the more you say a particular sound, the easier it becomes, because your brain creates pathways from the speech centers to the articulators so that they can move quickly to form a shape in the mouth.

By creating these neurological pathways and using them over and over again, the coordination and strength of the muscles in the jaw, lips, and tongue improve, ready for the production of the more difficult stage of producing consonant sounds. Say the vowels out loud and you will notice that your mouth stays open and quite still. Now say "shhh" out loud and you will notice that you move your lips, tongue, and jaw far more, which makes consonants much more complicated to master.

No wonder your little one finds it exciting to make these new noises. This experimentation is the workout for the main event! Just as a child can't jump without first learning to stand, walk, and run, a baby can't say words without going through the vowel and experimental noise phase. Which is why we need to go back to this crucial phase if your baby isn't babbling. Use my Top Tip techniques to encourage vowel sounds, eye contact, and experimental noises galore!

The following games will encourage your baby to make experimental noises.

**Top Tip Time** **Ready, set, go games**

- You'll need two rattles, one for you and one for your child. Say, "Ready, set . . . go," and make as much noise as you can with your rattle and with your voice. Then shout "Stop!" and see if your child is quiet. Repeat, repeat, repeat until a routine is established. When the routine is established, say, "Ready, set . . ." and wait. Wait for a sound or a movement from your little one as his way of saying "go" before you vigorously begin to shake the rattle again. The movement your baby makes might be an expression of excitement, such as a leg stiffening or a reach of the hand. A movement is likely to come before a sound but, as time goes by, wait for your baby to pair a movement and a sound (and, later, just make a sound) before you react.

- Build a tower of blocks or stacking cups. Say, "Up," as you build and encourage your child to say, "Up"—"uh. . . ." Then say, "Ready, set . . ." and wait in anticipation for them to make a noise or movement, before saying "go!" and knocking the tower down.

- Blow up a balloon without tying it and let it deflate. Then blow it up again without tying it and say, "Ready, set . . ." and wait to see if your child communicates to you for "go."

- Seat your child in a Bumbo seat or lay them on the floor. Take a ball or a toy car and say, "Ready, set . . ." and then, when they make a sound, roll the ball or wheel the car as fast as you can toward your child. For a car, make a raspberry noise, and for a ball, say "wee." Try singing this song: "Roll the ball, roll the ball, roll the ball to Libby. Libby has got the ball, now roll it back to me."

**Top Tip Time** **Anticipation games**

Now that your little one is making some experimental noises and beginning to engage, you are at the point where you can move forward with the art of turn-taking by expecting them to fully interact with you. In a way, you are putting a little bit of pressure on them to respond verbally—once they know a play routine well, they will anticipate a word or an action from you and you are anticipating a response from them. The key to this technique is in establishing a routine, so your little one knows exactly when they have to do an action or say a sound to receive their reward. The following are some games to try.

- Peekaboo is a great anticipation game. Your child will begin by passively watching your actions and then, eventually, will participate more actively by removing the cloth from their own face and attempting to say, "Boo."
- Put your phone to your ear and say, "Hello," then put the phone to your child's ear and wait as you look at them with an expectant face and nod to encourage them to make a noise.

### Songs and rhymes

Try the following simple anticipation songs and rhymes to encourage your child to engage and entice them to make some sounds or noises.

- Sing, "I can hear Jamie, running down the street, one two three, can you hear his feet? Ahh . . . ," then wait in anticipation for your child to make a sound. Once they do, finish the rhyme off with, "Run, run, run, run, run," moving their feet up and down.
- The old favorite "Pop Goes the Weasel" can be used as a fun anticipation game to tempt your child to communicate with you. When the song reaches the word *pop*, see if your child can attempt a sound in order to prompt you into making the "pop" noise.
- Lay your child on their back and hold their feet down on the ground. Sing the song "London Bridge" but change the words slightly by singing, "London bridge goes up, up, up," and lift their bottom up. Once they become familiar with the song, wait in anticipation for them to vocalize. Then you say, "Up, up, up."

# MY CHILD ISN'T ENGAGING VERBALLY BUT IS ATTEMPTING SOME ACTIONS TO SONGS—LET'S TRY SOME SIGNING! 4 SIMPLE SIGNS TO TRY

Now that your little one is experimenting with their mouth and hands in songs, encourage them to experiment with their hands as a means to express themself—let's start signing (see page 71).

All babies learn gestures or signs before they learn to say words (for example, waving for "bye-bye" or arms up for "lift me up") so encourage your child to use these signs and others, and this will encourage them to learn to intentionally communicate their wants and needs. The success of baby signing is because if you sign, you provide visual information and words simultaneously. Signs are considered to be visual cues, which reinforce spoken language, so your little one will grasp language more quickly. Signing can be used with all children, and SLPs are passionate about it because it gives a child a means to communicate way before they can actually speak, inspiring them to expand their communication skills more rapidly.

There are a few signs that I recommend you try to introduce as early as possible—these are signs that you will probably be using without even realizing because they are almost an extension of natural gestures. These are "bye-bye," "up," "finished," and "more."

The four signs shown below can be incorporated easily into your everyday routine—"up" each time you lift up your child, "finished" at bath time or when they've finished their milk, and "more" each time they are having fun playing a game with you.

Noticing how your little one engages and connects with you at such an early age is crucially important when it comes to learning language a little later on. Try to make the golden rules of Special Time and Say What You See a habit that you don't even need to think about, so the building blocks for learning to talk are firmly in place as your child starts their journey toward becoming a chatty child!

Chapter 3

# What to do when . . . your baby isn't babbling

We learned in chapter 2 that the seemingly meaningless squeals, screeches, and cooing noises (called pre-babble) your child makes are the crucial building blocks from which they'll begin to form babble sounds, then words, and ultimately sentences. If you've noticed a delay in this area already, you've hopefully been tuning in and engaging with your child to encourage them to make experimental noises. You might even have started to reward their attempts to communicate, using the Top Tips for Talking (playing peekaboo; Ready, Set, Go; and other Top Tip Time games). Your little one is starting to understand that communication is a two-way process.

A young child's innate need to socially interact with others never ceases to amaze and delight me. Generally children become really sociable at a young age, craving human contact and attention. You might spot your little one having great fun engaging strangers—for instance, by making eye contact in a supermarket aisle or across the table in a restaurant—all with the aim of getting a rewarding response such as a smile or a comment from another person. The tricky thing is, if your child has a delay, they may still want to do this when they're much older, and other people are less likely to respond to an older child—so you have to encourage this by smiling at the stranger yourself as an icebreaker.

Your little one might want to "play" with and take notice of their little friends, too, and will chase them, crawling or toddling, wanting to pull their hair, reach for them, show them something, or even try to start a "conversation." Again, this is accepted when the child is younger but not so much when the perception is that they should know better. It's tough. And that's when parents begin to feel like others are looking at them in a disapproving way, and of course parental guilt isn't too far behind.

You may also find that there are periods of time where the stages of child development are obvious to parents—for instance during the 6-to-12-month phase, children learn to sit, crawl, stand, feed themselves, etc., in a short space of time—but other phases are less obvious, as with communication skills in which you may not see obvious changes. But I can assure you that lots of things are happening under the surface that are crucial to speech and communication.

Let's start, though, by looking at how a child's "pre-babble" develops into "babble."

## WHAT IS BABBLE?

Before a child starts to babble, they will have been through a pre-babble phase during which they begin to experiment with sounds, random noises, and some vowel sounds (as described in chapter 2). During the babble phase, you will start hearing their first consonant sounds—"p," "b," "m" and "w," and then, later, "d" and "g"—consonant sounds appear in a predetermined developmental order.

Babble is the sound made when the same consonant sound is added to a familiar vowel noise; for example, "ba-ba" or "goo-goo." This is known as reduplicated babble and might appear as early as 5 months old. It then moves to adding two consonant sounds together, such as "mu-bu" or "du-wu"—known as varie-gated babble, which might appear by about 8 to 9 months. By 10 months the babble might become more elaborate, reaching four or five syllables and varied tones. This is known as conversation-al babble, or gibberish—"goo-eee-yah," "bay-me-ooo-du," "ka-da-bu-ba." This stage occurs just before a child starts to attempt proper words.

Obviously, as most real words are made up of consonants and vowels, being able to make babble sounds is a crucial step on the journey toward using real words.

We had real problems with our daughter, Jess, during the bab-ble phase. She got into a habit of saying "buh-guh," which, un-fortunately, sounded very much like the British curse word "bug-ger"—obviously, not a great first word. She'd say it at the most inappropriate times—when my husband's great-aunt came to stay, when visiting the dentist, and continuously when we put her on the phone to say hi to her grandparents. The trouble was, it got a lot of attention and Jess knew it. My dad and father-in-law would continuously repeat it and even initiate a conversation with, "Buh-guh, buh-guh." We had to draw a line when things got worse and she started saying, "Hiya, buh-guh." So I began not reacting at all and insisting that no one else do so, either. Sooner or later it disappeared to make way for a second round of swearing in teen-age years!

This is how babbling and, later, real words begin—they all happen accidentally. A baby might say "mu-mu" in play but is rewarded with a response along the lines of, "Oh, yes—mu-mu, mu-mu," and then they want to say it again because they enjoyed the reaction they got. If an experimental noise or babble sound is not rewarded, after some time it'll fade away. So, bye-bye beastly "buh-guh"! Thus, we have to create as many opportunities as we can for children to practice saying random sounds in situations where we're interacting with them so we can reward them.

# What's happening in your baby's brain?

While your baby is busy babbling, a vast network of neurological pathways is being created in their brain, and the reason babies babble in such a repetitive way is that it helps the brain to generate and practice using these neural pathways. (Just to remind you, these are the connections that run from brain to mouth to enable speaking.) So, the more a baby says "ba-ba-ba," the more deep-rooted and robust the neural pathways for making that sound will be.

Newborns arrive with a limited amount of neurological wiring. There are some very basic connections in terms of vision, hearing, and the other senses. But in the cerebellum (the "little brain" tucked under the main hemispheres), nothing is wired at all; the hardware is in place and ready to "wire up," but it requires real-life experiences and human interactions so that the cells can join together, creating a network of neurological pathways that will become the foundation for thinking and reasoning, language, and social and emotional behaviors.

Let's think about this in terms of understanding. Each time you say the word *Nana* when your child is looking at Nana, those links in the brain are getting stronger and stronger and will become so well established that, when you say "Nana" and she's not visibly there, your child will still know who you are talking about. Eventually, the pathways will run from the brain down to the articulators (the jaw, lips, and tongue that help us to form sounds that become words) so that, in time, your child will try and say, "Nana." So, whenever you communicate with your child you are helping develop their thinking and concentration skills. (These skills fall under the heading of cognitive skills, which are perception, thinking, and learning skills.)

Early experiences and interactions with a responsive and attentive caregiver are the most critical factors in a child's brain development—from birth, the brain rapidly creates these connections that form our habits, thoughts, consciousness, memories, and reasoning.

If you want to learn more about this, look at the attachment theory section in Sue Gerhardt's bestselling book *Why Love Matters*.

This is why the brain of a 3-year-old is supposedly two and a half times more active than an adult's. During the first three years of life, a child's brain builds an estimated one thousand trillion links through the experiences they encounter. Babies are constantly looking, listening, and moving, so just imagine all the experiences they are having and all the connections their brains are making.

It's so clever, isn't it? So when I see a toddler or child who has a speech or language delay in my clinic, one of the first questions I ask the parent is, "Did your child go through a babble phase?" as it is integral to later speech and language development. The good news is that there are many games you can play to encourage the babble stage in all its glory.

**Top Tip Time** **Encouraging babble**

Just as babble is made up of a chain of repetitive noises, it is really important to repeat the same games over and over again so your little one will continuously hear the same words and sounds. Even though it might seem boring to you, babies enjoy endlessly hearing the same fun, lyrical words being used repetitively as it helps them to build neural pathways. Below are some games to try:

- Copy the noises your child makes. Try to develop a turn-taking conversation—the child says "du" and you say "du." Wait and see if they say anything else. If so, repeat it. Then you say a simple babble sound and wait for your child to say something. They won't be able to say your sound immediately, but if you repeat this activity over and over again, a little copycat will, one hopes, be brought to life.

- Copy each other's noises in the mirror. Make sure you can both see each other's face and your child will have a better chance of modeling your mouth shapes.

- Give your little one a toy phone or Toobaloo in order to encourage them to babble. A Toobaloo looks like an old-fashioned phone handset and encourages children to talk by amplifying the sounds into their ears as they talk into it. This motivates children to say more.

- Use puppets to generate noises by making the puppet say a stream of babble sounds in a conversational way, such as "ah ba-ba-ba-ba-ba." Stop and wait for them to join in. Then try again with "ah ba-ba"—be as animated as possible. If you don't have a puppet, make one from a sock.

- Make a babble bag, a set of toys that encourage your child to babble—for example, a pretend mobile phone, a talking toucan (a bird that repeats the noises you say), a microphone, a mirror, a noisy book, a paper-towel tube that makes an echo when you speak down it, a couple of animals that make distinct noises—such as "moo-moo" or "woof-woof"—a car (so you can say "brum-brum") and two puppets to experiment with.

## IS YOUR CHILD BECOMING SUPER INTERACTIVE AND EASY TO ENGAGE WITH?

As babies move from the pre-babble phase to the babble phase, their nonverbal communication also tends to boom with nodding, waving, babbling, clapping, signing, pointing, and book sharing becoming huge fun (you'll be amazed at how infectious your child's giggle is). Singing and playing games like "Round and Round the Garden" are endlessly entertaining—for you and your little one. And they'll want the fun to go on and on—peekaboo can last an eternity and simply never seems to get boring or repetitive.

This is when the well-worn speech therapy phrase "Language develops through play" really comes alive. Our children love to play and will hopefully seek out their best playmate (that's you, by the way) to play with. Their personality and sense of humor will start to shine through, and you're in store for endless hours of fun. But again I want to emphasize that if this is not the case, there are lots of fun games and activities you can do with your child to encourage them.

**Top Tip Time** **Early interaction**

The following games and activities will help to boost your child's engagement with you, as well as their communication and their interactivity.

Try interactive songs or clapping games, such as "Pat-a-Cake." The crucial thing about these games is that you are communicating with your child at their language level and expecting them to join in with you (read more information on singing, page 64).

## CLASSIC CLAPPING GAMES

Say the following nursery rhyme to your little one, adding some clapping where indicated.

*Pat a cake, pat a cake* [clap hands], *baker's man,*
*Make me a cake as fast as you can.*
*Roll it* [move your hands in a rolling motion] *and pat it* [pat your knees] *and mark it with a B,*
*And put it in the oven for baby and me [point to baby and point to yourself],*
*For baby and me, for baby and me* [continue pointing],
*Yes, there will be plenty for baby and me* [continue pointing].

Sit your child on your lap and sing, "We're going up and down and up and down and side to side and side to side and round and round and round and round and over the deep blue sea." (Move your child around according to the words.)

Lay your child on their back and say the following rhyme.

*Knock at the door* (Knock on their forehead)
*Peep in* (Make their eyes open slightly wider)
*Lift up the latch* (Push up their nose)
*Walk in* (Pretend to put your finger in their mouth)
*Take a chair* (Pinch their left cheek)
*Sit down there* (Pinch their right cheek)
*How do you do today?* (Make their chin go up and down)

# Giving your little one a reason to communicate

Children need a reason, an opportunity, and a means to communicate. I've always found the following list of reasons why a child might try to communicate very helpful for making parents aware of all the instances when their newborn to 4-year-old might be communicating, particularly when they might be using only their voice rather than real words to do so. Once you know what motivates your little one to want to communicate, whether it be as a request or a protest, you can provide many opportunities during your day to encourage them to tell you their wishes.

Take your cue from the situations below,[1] then watch and wait to see how your child responds.

- Responding: "Yes"/"Bye-bye." Do they use their voice to respond to other people?
- Requesting: "Cookie"/"More." Do they use their voice when they want something?
- Protesting/refusing: "No!"/"Go away." Or when they don't want something?
- For getting attention: Mummmmy!"
- For making comments: "Look!"/"Big bus."
- To give information: "Me fall down."
- For seeking information: "What's that?"/"Where's Daddy gone?"
- Thinking and planning: "After dinner"/"Bath time."
- And sharing ideas: "Let's go park!"/"I like ice cream."

# HELP YOUR CHILD LEARN TO LISTEN

## Developing the skill of listening

In order for a child to acquire the words they eventually want to say, they first have to learn to listen to language, so they can recognize, remember, and repeat the words we model for them. Listening is fundamental to a child's ability to transition from babbling to attempting first words.

You might think that listening is a skill that just comes naturally, but listening is different from hearing. A child may have normal hearing but might find it difficult to listen, so we have to teach them to listen.

If your child has a good ability to stay calm and focused, they'll have good listening, which means that they will stay with a game or an activity for longer, allowing them more time to think about it and learn the words that are associated with the game. Thinking and concentration come under the category of cognitive skills and, therefore, the more you practice these skills, the higher the chance of realizing your intellectual potential.

## CASE STUDY: FINN LEARNS TO LISTEN

One of the tricky things about my job is when I see something in a friend's child that I think could be helped with a couple of Top Tips. This happened with Finn, who was 11 months old. He rarely said anything and nobody seemed at all concerned. He had three older siblings, all under the age of 6, and lived in a busy, noisy house. He was a sociable boy who smiled a lot and gave great eye contact but rarely spoke. One day I plucked up the courage and said, "Finn is quite quiet when we meet up. Is it because he's mesmerized by all the others running around?" The answer was, "Umm, I hadn't really noticed. I suppose it must be." Me: "Does he say a lot at home?" Answer: "Yes, I think so." Me: "Oh, that's good." End of conversation.

Two nights later, the phone rang. "Hi, Nic; it's Gaynor. I was thinking about what you said the other day about Finn being quiet, and I've noticed that he hardly tries to say a word at home."

"Well, what does he say?" I asked. Answer: "He copies the dog barking and makes a loud 'ahh' sound when the others are making a lot of noise." Hmm, I was right: There was a problem. So, here's what we did.

- First, I referred Finn for a hearing test. His hearing was slightly down on both sides and he had a history of ear infections in both ears, suggesting that at one point, maybe a critical point in his development, he would have found it difficult to hear and perhaps, even now, his hearing was fluctuating.

- Every day we gave Finn 10 minutes of Special Time when he had a bit of one-on-one time with Mum, Dad, or me, with as little background noise as possible. We had to train his ears to listen—this may have been because during one of the periods when his hearing was low, he got into a habit of not listening because there was nothing to listen to. You have to hear sounds in order to try to copy them!

- Each Special Time started with the adult saying, "Shhh," and then waiting for a sound to listen to. (One day, I set off the alarm on my cell phone and hid it under the bed just so that he would hear a different sound from those sounds his siblings were making!)

- We made a babble bag (page 55).

- We also had a sound sack for Finn to play with. This consisted of a bag of objects that we could use as props, waving them around as we made specific speech-sound noises that suited each animal and are used in the English language—for example, a monkey ("ooo-ooo-ooo"), a mouse ("eee-eee-eee"), a teddy ("ahhh"), a train ("ch-ch") and a rabbit ("ff-ff"). It was much easier to gather the objects together, so whenever we had 5 minutes we could just pull something out of the box and get started right away.

Within a month, Finn was making a much wider range of noises and everyone was a lot less worried. He seemed a little more content, too, and easier to engage with. He continued to make good progress and didn't need any official speech therapy support in the end.

## The benefit of cause-and-effect games

I encourage all my families to play with cause-and-effect toys—these are games with which an action from the child results in an exciting reward for all. So, you might push a button and an animal pops up, squeeze teddy's tummy and he starts to sing, clap your hands and puppy starts dancing, pull a string and the duck quacks, and so on.

Why am I such a fan? Think about communication. If a child understands the concept that their actions will make something happen, then they will be likely to attempt a word to get what they want. In other words, they realize that if they say, "More," Daddy will tickle them again, or if they say, "Drink," they'll get a drink, and if they say, "Duck," Mummy starts singing "Five Little Ducks." This is a learned behavior from playing with cause-and-effect toys.

Try not to predict your child's needs and wants all the time. For instance, if at 10:30 AM your child usually gets a drink and a cookie, wait until 10:45 AM and see if they communicate what they want by pulling you, pointing, signing, or trying to attempt the word. Remember—communication can be verbal and nonverbal during this phase.

**Top Tip Time** **Learning to listen and concentrate**

Listening for language can be very difficult when there is a constant background noise such as the TV or the radio—you might want to look back at my Top Tips for Talking in chapter 1 about setting the scene, as all the same rules still apply. The games below start with the most basic listening skills and get more complex, so try to run through them in order.

### Make lots of noise as you play
Shake keys and rattles, bang drums and pots, or play together and copy each other.

## Noise, then no noise

- I love rainmakers or rain sticks, those toys full of tiny beads that you tip up to hear the sound of rain. You need to say, "Listen to the rain, raining, raining, raining. Stop."
- Is the washing machine on? Listen to the sound of it spinning and then stopping.
- Try presenting your child with an array of containers, some that are filled and some that are empty. Try using dry rice or pasta, a toy car, and frozen peas to put into the containers. I sometimes walk around the garden with a plastic takeout container and, when my daughter looks at something, I will put it into the box and shake it to see what sound it makes.

There's a great song for which you will need something very noisy such as bells or metal tins full of metal spoons. It goes like this.

> *Shake and shake and shake and stop [make the silence last a while, then repeat three times].*
> *And then we're going to shake some more—shake, shake, shake, shake, shake, shake, stop.*

## Listen to noises in your environment

- Go outside and say, "Shhhhhhh," and wait . . . what do you hear? Cars, birds, roadwork, dogs, trains, leaves blowing in the trees, a helicopter, or perhaps silence? Try to verbalize what you hear.
- If there is a sound in your house (for example, the vacuum cleaner, the washing machine, dishwasher, doorbell, phone, or tea kettle boiling), draw your child's attention to it. Say, "Shhhh," again before you draw their attention to the noise, so that they know that they have to listen.

## Where is the noise coming from?

First of all, turn off other noises like the TV or radio. Now, find a noisy toy or an alarm clock and play with the noise so your child becomes accustomed to the sound it makes. Then, when they are not looking, put the toy behind them and say, "Where has the clock gone?" Encourage your child to look for it. Once you have done this a few times, hide the toy somewhere farther afield (under a table, in a cardboard box, or behind the sofa, for example) so that your child can crawl and find it.

## Symbolic noises

- Listen together to things that make a distinctive noise—for example, vehicles (cars, trains, emergency service vehicles, and airplanes) or different kinds of animals.
- Toy animals are also great for this game—hold two up and say one animal's noise, watching to see if your child looks to or reaches for the correct one. If the animal doesn't have a specific noise, like a rabbit, I usually give the animal a speech-sound noise such as "ff, ff, ff" (biting your lip with your front teeth). For giraffe I always say, "j, j, j" (bear in mind that giraffe starts with a "j" sound rather than a "g" sound).
- Favorite toys can also be given their own noise—with dolls I usually say, "Ahh," when they get a cuddle, and for ball it's "b, b, b, b"—intentionally the first "sound" of the word.
- Make a babble bag. Put the noisy objects your child likes the most into a bag. Besides the suggestions given previously, you could add a cuddly toy with a large nose to press and say, "Beep-beep," a cat that says "Meow," or a fire engine that goes "nee-nor." Pull them out one at a time, and when you look at these objects, say their sounds over and over again. Help your child to listen to and learn the noises. Say the sound "brum-brum" while the car is moving and go silent when it stops. You could also try putting a mirror in the bag to encourage your child to say the sounds and to look at the way their mouth moves as they say them.
- Make a sound sack (see pages 59 and 139).

## Listening to voices

- Hide behind the curtains, behind the sofa, under a blanket, under the table, or behind the door, then call your child's name. Can they find where you are hidden? Say, "Peekaboo" when they find you. (Warning: This game can go on for hours!)

- Ready, set, go games—get them to knock down a tower of blocks or roll a ball in response to your saying, "Go." Try tickling them after you say, "Go," and so on.
- Sing a familiar song and then wait for your child to react when you pause before the key word—for example, "If you see a crocodile, don't forget to . . . scream . . . argh!" (Read more on why children love songs so much, page 64.)

## Babies can lip-read

Babies don't learn to talk just from hearing sounds. New research suggests they're lip-readers, too. Scientists in Florida have discovered that, starting around the age of 6 months, babies begin shifting from the intent eye gaze of early infancy to studying mouths when people talk to them. "The baby, in order to imitate you, has to figure out how to shape their lips to make that particular sound they're hearing," explains developmental psychologist David Lewkowicz of Florida Atlantic University, who led the study.[2]

Apparently, it doesn't take babies too long to absorb the movements that match basic sounds. By their first birthday, babies start shifting back to looking you in the eye again—unless they hear the unfamiliar sounds of a foreign language. Then, they stick with lip-reading for a bit longer.

This research confirms just how important it is to get down to your child's level and have quality face-to-face time with them (as opposed to sitting them in front of the latest baby YouTube video) when it comes to speech development.

## SINGING

Parents have been singing songs and lullabies to their children for thousands of years, passing down the rhymes through many generations. Children love songs and rhymes—have you ever noticed that when a song from a commercial comes on the TV or when you put music on in the car, your child stops and calms down? And for good reason—babies love the familiarity of songs and, because of the continuous repetition of the same words, they find learning words through songs easier than learning words through spoken words. A recent study of brain scans at Johns Hopkins showed that when people hear music, the language center in the brain lights up.[3] Even more reason to start singing.

The same applies to adults—a tune might come on the radio that you haven't heard for years but you'll find yourself singing along because the words come back to you as soon as you hear the music. Having a tune and a rhythm helps you to remember the words.

So, this is why we have a section on singing here when perhaps you might have thought that, by the age of 6 months plus, you'd have stopped singing lullabies to your baby and would have moved on to speaking. In fact, the opposite is true—I encourage the parents who visit my clinic to keep singing to their children for years!

---

### MY FAVORITE SONGS FOR EVERYDAY ROUTINES

Choose short and simple songs that are easy for your child to learn and remember. Here are some of my favorites.

- Whenever you see your child go from sitting to standing, sing the following words to the tune of "Step in Time."

*Jess is standing, standing tall*
*Jess is standing, standing tall*

---

*Jess is standing, Jess is standing*
*Jess is standing, standing tall!*

- Try tidying up singing the following words to the tune of "The Farmer in the Dell."

*It's time to tidy up, it's time to tidy up.*
*Tidy up, tidy up,*
*It's time to tidy up.*

- Carry out your morning routine while singing "This Is the Way We Wash Our Hands" (wash our face/brush our teeth).

- For teaching body parts, try the old classic "Head, Shoulders, Knees, and Toes," or another song I like is "Put Your Finger on Your Nose," which you sing to the tune of "If You're Happy and You Know It." The lyrics are here.

*Put your finger on your nose, on your nose,*
*Put your finger on your nose, on your nose,*
*Put your finger on your nose,*
*That's where the cold wind blows.*
*Put your finger on your nose, on your nose,*
*Put your finger on your ear, on your ear,*
*Put your finger on your ear, on your ear,*
*Put your finger on your ear,*
*And leave it there all year.*
*Put your finger on your ear, on your ear,*
*Put your finger on your knee, on your knee,*
*Put your finger on your knee, on your knee,*
*Put your finger on your knee,*
*We're as happy as can be.*
*Put your finger on your knee, on your knee,*
*Put your fingers all together, all together,*
*Put your fingers all together, all together,*
*Put your fingers all together,*
*And pray for better weather.*
*Put your fingers all together, all together.*

**Top Tip Time** **Learning through singing**

You are probably going to have to sing "Twinkle, Twinkle, Little Star" and other nursery rhymes hundreds of times with your little one, so I figure you may as well learn how to get the most out of it! Below, I'll give you some pointers. If you think your child really enjoys the song and wants more, encourage them to say and/or sign "more" before you sing again.

### Go slow and praise

Look expectantly at your child to encourage them to join in when singing. This will help them to make sense of the words and enable them to participate in their own way. So, you might hear them trying to join in the "quack, quack, quack" part of "Five Little Ducks," scream when they "see" the crocodile in "Row, Row, Row Your Boat," or indicate that they want more of the song "Bouncing Up and Down in My Little Red Wagon" by bouncing.

Just don't go so slowly that the rhythm is lost, or that your child's attention is compromised. Try to focus on one song for 5 minutes a day.

### Stress and repeat words

Choose songs in which the same words appear time and time again (for example, "Five Little Ducks" offers plenty of repetition). This enables you to stress that word time and time again. There is a reason why children love the rhyme "The Wheels on the Bus"— the lyrics are simple and repetitive and the word *bus* gets repeated time and time again.

### Sing songs with actions and signs for the words

This helps the child to understand the meaning. Two of my favorite action songs are "Itsy Bitsy Spider" (where you use your hands to show a spider climbing up the waterspout, then being washed down, and then fan your hands to show the sun coming out) and "Twinkle, Twinkle, Little Star" (where you wiggle your fingers to show a sparkling star above your child's head and form a triangle shape to show a diamond in the sky).

## Encourage participation

Decide what your child should do to take part—for example, clap, sign (read more information on signing, page 71), or sing a word—and begin to teach the song with the aim that they will start filling in the gaps. Just as with anticipation games, when you pause during the song (ideally, before the key word or action), stop, look at your child expectantly (sometimes for a time that feels far too long for an adult, say, 5 to 8 seconds) and wait for your child to respond in some way. This won't be the real word initially, but, instead, a look, body movement or sound suggesting that they know they have to say or do something at this time. Remember to give lots of praise.

If your goal is to get your little one participating with a clap or a sign (for example, in "If You're Happy and You Know It"), take their hands in your own and help to move them appropriately, then move your hands farther down their arms so that they move their hands alone, then simply push their elbows to show that you are expecting them to clap.

If you want your little one to contribute a particular word, then choose the word carefully—the word at the end of the phrase often stands out, or the word that is frequently repeated. Slow down before the word appears and look expectantly at your child, in anticipation, then say the word yourself if they don't say it, so that you don't lose the thread of the song. Initially, you'll encourage them to say one word, then increase it to two, three, then more words.

## ACTIVITIES FOR VERY EARLY LANGUAGE DEVELOPMENT

Research at the University of Dundee found that activities including singing nursery rhymes, sharing books, and reminiscing (such as looking at photo albums) all promote language development.[4] Researchers found that repetition is also important—if children are learning new words, they remember them better if they look at them again and again in the same book.

# IS YOUR CHILD POINTING AND USING GESTURES?

From as young as 7 months, but usually around 8 to 11 months, a child starts to use natural gestures such as waving, reaching, and pointing to communicate. This suggests that coordinating the movements of our hands is far easier than coordinating the lungs and articulators in order to speak. So, try to make the most of your child's ability to use their hands functionally and teach them to communicate with them!

## Pointing

Did you know that we are the only animals that point? Well, I suppose most animals have paws, which makes it a bit tricky, but even chimps raised with humans rarely point and never point to other chimps.

That must mean that it's a very intelligent thing to do—it draws other people's attention to what *you* want them to focus on, even when that object is some distance away. It might be as a request for something, or to demonstrate your interest in something to another person. When two people are focusing on the same thing, it's known as joint attention and, for good communication, it's a very important skill to acquire. Amazingly, little ones who can't talk will even point to each other as a form of communication! Our children will understand a point long before they start to point themselves and will turn their heads or look to respond.

You might see your little one point to food they want in the fridge, to people they want to be picked up by, to pictures in a book that they want you to name for them or to the door if they want to leave. But it is tricky and some children take a little while to master this skill.

Sometimes, the point may be accompanied by a sound but, often, it is not. And a little one usually looks at you before and after the point, to check that their message has been received. (This is different from a child on the autistic spectrum, who may reach instead of point and do so when nobody is around to receive their attempts to communicate, not understanding the concept of joint attention.)

With just a tiny flip of an index finger, a whole new world opens up for your little one. They'll point and, instinctively, you'll look at the object and name it. This could happen time and time again as they learn the words and store them in their word bank, ready to use in a few months' time.

## POINTING AND THE ACQUISITION OF SPEECH

This simple gesture is so important that the rate of speech acquisition is correlated with the onset of pointing. Luigia Camaioni, of the University of Rome, found that the earlier babies begin to point, the more words they know at 20 months of age.[5]

**Top Tip Time** **Pointing games and activities**

- First, establish whether or not your child understands the purpose of pointing. To find this out, direct their attention with your finger to an object within close range. Don't point to an object that is making noise (a radio, television, telephone, and so on) because they may follow the noise rather than your finger's aim. Do they look at the object to which you are pointing? Or are they looking at your finger? How do they respond? Then establish whether they understand the function of their own point. Take your child's finger and use it to point to something—do they look at where their finger points to? If not, use lots of tactile books, such as the Touch and Feel series and encourage them to point to pictures that will provide sensory feedback and to look where their finger is placed.

- It's important for your child to understand the purpose of pointing, because they may not attempt to point themselves. So, if you feel they don't understand the function of pointing, start pointing all the time at things in your environment. Point to things that are in close range, like facial features, then toys that are just beyond your finger, then things that are slightly farther away, like a bus or a police car.

- Once you think your child understands what's going on when you point, try singing the following finger-based songs: "Where Is Thumbkin?," "The Finger Family Song," and "Head, Shoulders, Knees, and Toes." This will encourage them to isolate one finger.

- Play with toys that encourage fine motor development (intricate movements with the fingers), such as an old-fashioned phone, a pop-up game, or even, dare I say it, an iPad or an iPhone, for which isolating one finger is integral. Scatter cereal such as Cheerios on the table and encourage your child to eat it by picking the pieces up using a pincer grip (finger and thumb together). Once they can isolate one finger to form a pincer grip, mold their hand into a pointing shape—you may have to put your own finger in their palm so that they can grip something in order to hold their other three fingers down.

- Put something you know your child loves just out of their reach and, when they reach for it, give it. Then try it again.

Adjust your child's hand into the pointing position for the required object. Repeat this again and again using a range of very motivating objects.

## Signing

So, seeing as your child is naturally beginning to use gestures, why don't we teach them more gestures and start basic signing? You could enroll in a baby signing course with your little one or buy a simple baby signing book, such as *Baby Signs* by Joy Allen.

### Signing does not hold back speech development

Often, when parents come into my clinic with their children and I encourage them to start signing as part of the therapy process, they object, saying that they want their child to talk, not sign. There is a common misconception that learning to sign hinders talking but, in actual fact, this couldn't be further from the truth, and I am very happy to bust the myth, right here, right now.

If you think about a child's developmental stages, children naturally use gestures before they speak. For example, they wave, clap, and reach their arms up to show they want to be picked up. Making these gestures doesn't stop them from eventually saying those words; it merely helps them to communicate their needs and wants when they don't yet have the words to express themselves. Once the word is learned, the gesture or sign should fade away.

Another way to think about the relationship between signing and speech is in terms of crawling and walking. We all accept it's good for children to go through a phase of crawling because it helps them to develop the motor skills that they need to master in order to begin walking. But when they start to walk, they stop crawling fairly quickly. So, crawling is a natural step toward walking, just as using gesture and sign is a natural phase to pass through before talking begins. I assure you, signing will actively encourage your child's first words, not hold them back.

## The benefits of signing

- **It's easier to sign than it is to speak.** Research into language development has shown that signs and gestures are easier to learn than spoken words. After all, as I showed you in chapter 1, speech is a very complex process—it involves the coordination of breath, vocal cords, the jaw, the lips, and the tongue and an explosion of brain cell activation. For your child to utter just one word, they may have to coordinate five or more mouth shapes. By contrast, a gesture requires far simpler brain and body processes because, at this stage of development, babies have better visual and physical than verbal skills.

- **Children can see the signs they are making.** To make things even harder, when a little one attempts a word, they cannot see if they are getting it right because they can't see their own mouth. This, in my opinion, is where signing excels. A child can watch their arms, hands, and fingers moving when they wave or point "up," which makes the motion easier to control. You can also physically assist a child to sign, further reinforcing the sign and its meaning, but you can't do this with speech.

- **Signing helps parents simplify their language.** Given that most parents master signs at the same time as their child, signing also helps the talker to simplify and slow down his or her language, enabling the child to hear a clear model for language. For example, an adult might say, "Do you want another apple?" but if you only know the signs for "more" and "apple," you are more likely to say, "More apple?"

- **Signing also helps the talker to use consistent language.** The signer will only know a certain number of signs, so they will tend to use consistent signs for the same word. So, without a sign an adult might say, "Do you want din-din?," "Are you hungry?," or "It's snack time!," but if the parent only knows the sign for "eat," your child will usually say, "Let's eat."

And, as you hopefully have already learned, repeating the same word or sign constantly is the best way for your little one to learn what this word means, and the context in which to use it. Once they understand, they will try to say it.

- **Signing reduces frustration.** All children's level of understanding and thinking is greater than their ability to express themselves verbally. In other words, by 10 months of age, your little one should be able to understand some single words like "Daddy," "bath," "drink," or "milk," but won't be able to say them. Imagine how frustrating this must be— just think about being in a country where you don't speak the language, but you know exactly what you want to say and you just can't get your message across.

  Children often become frustrated when they can't express themselves. Young children may communicate this through behaviors such as tantrums, screaming, and kicking. By using signs, we are helping them to communicate in a more acceptable way.

- **Signing boosts understanding.** Signs also add extra information to the child's attempts to speak, helping parents to understand what their child is trying to say. When a child first starts talking, they may use the same utterance for many different words. For example, "buh" may mean "bus," "book," "boo," etc., but if the word attempt is made alongside the sign, then the listener will always know what the word is.

- **Signing helps concentration and listening.** Children find it easier to focus on things that are moving, so when your hands are moving to create signs your child is more likely to look and listen. If two people stand next to each other and say the same sentence, but one is gesturing and the other just talks, a child will most definitely be looking at the person moving their hands. Think about how your eyes are drawn to a flickering fire or a moving TV screen, even though you are not particularly concentrating on it.

- **Don't be intimidated by the thought of learning sign language.** Some parents panic at the thought of learning to sign, as they think they have to master a full signing vocabulary, but I want to reassure you that you only need to master the basics. And the good news is that signs are usually pretty logical and often look like the words they mean. For example, the sign for "car" is like driving a car where you pretend you are turning a steering wheel.

In fact, many are so obvious, you actually already do them without even realizing. How often have you signaled to others that they should call you by simply pretending that you are holding a phone to your ear? This is the sign for "phone"! And guess what—the sign for "goodbye" is waving.

## Signing rules

- Gain the child's attention and make eye contact before you sign.
- Always accompany signs with clear speech and facial expressions.
- Only sign key words—words that are important for the meaning. Keep your sentences, and therefore your signs, simple and short. So, rather than saying, "It's ten o'clock. Let's get your coat on and go swimming," it's far better to say and sign, "Swimming time!"
- Reward and praise any attempt to communicate.
- Signs need to be used by everyone in the child's environment, so encourage your partner, older siblings, Granny and Grandpa, and the caregiver to get involved! Ask your local SLP about free signing courses and encourage as many people as possible to attend. If you can get a group of willing candidates together, I'm sure the SLP will train your self-assembled group if you ask kindly!
- Keep signing even if, at first, your child doesn't attempt to sign back.
- Many children need hand-over-hand help to start signing, in which you assist your child by taking their hands to mold them into the right position for the sign, just as you take your child's hands when you encourage them to wave.
- Remember that signing skills are developed over time through practice and repetition. The time it takes depends on the age of the child and the frequency at which they are being signed to.

- Remember to have fun. Signing shouldn't feel like a chore or something extra to add to your to-do list. The more you do it, the more it'll feel like second nature, part of the way you communicate.

## CASE STUDY: EVIE GETS SIGNING

Beckie is an SLP friend of mine who has two daughters, Evie and Leila. She is a great advocate for baby-led weaning and she also taught her daughters to sign.

Beckie started signing with Evie when she was 6½ months old. In hindsight, she thinks this is too young for most nonprofessional folk as Evie didn't sign back until about 10 months and, because it took so long, most parents would have given up long before, since there was no immediate gratification.

Beckie started with only a handful of signs that were meaningful for Evie—"more," "finished," "eat," and "drink"— and she bombarded her with them during as many everyday activities as possible. Once Evie started signing back, Beckie really stepped up the pace and often used the hand-over-hand method (see previous page) to encourage Evie with new signs. By 14 months, Evie had a spoken vocabulary of 20 words and a signed vocabulary of 20 words. Interestingly, there were only two words that Evie could both sign and say. That's forty words by 14 months—amazing!

It seems that the area in which Evie really gained the most benefit from Beckie's signing was in her understanding. She had fantastic understanding and that makes perfect sense— the spoken words were backed up visually by signs to support learning. And, because she had such good understanding at an earlier age, she had a wider vocabulary at an earlier age.

# DOES YOUR LITTLE ONE SHOW SOME LEVEL OF UNDERSTANDING?

At around 9 months, a baby's memory begins to build dramatically and they will begin to understand more of what you say. Remember—children usually understand words long before they actually use them.

You'll know your child understands you when you say, "Daddy's home!," for instance, and your little one looks at the door, or when you say, "Ball," and they crawl right to it, or when you say, "Kiss," and they bring their head toward yours for a kiss. By this stage, your little one should respond well to their own name and should look up (or at least pause) when you say a firm "stop." They may even respond to little phrases like "come here," "bye-bye," "give me," "blow kiss," and so on.

You will notice that your baby's understanding is improving every day and, by the age of 1, they might be able to understand as many as 50 words!

**Top Tip Time**  **Boosting understanding**

### Keep what you say short and simple

Talk about toys and read stories using single words or very short phrases. If your child can only understand single words or very short phrases, such as "Finished" or "What's that?," then you must speak to them at this level so that they remember the words, understand them, and then start to copy them.

### Use repetitive language and keep your routine language consistent

If you tend to say, "Wash your face," repeat this phrase rather than changing it to "Wipe your mouth" after the next meal. When you go into your little one's room in the morning, try to run through routine language, saying, "Hello, gorgeous. Did you have a lovely sleep? Coming up? Ah, up to Mummy for a cuddle. Open the curtains. Good morning, trees, good morning, garden, good morning, swing." Similarly, at bedtime, use consistent language as sleep time cues, such as "Night-night, Erik. Night-night, Teddy. Sleep tight. Say 'Night-night, Mummy.' See you in the morning."

### Talk about the here and now

This allows your little one to get immediate feedback about what is happening in their life (refer back to Say What You See, pages 24–26).

### Remember the importance of encouraging your child to focus on you

When you say something, ensure you gain your child's attention before you speak.

### Use gestures and signs

Use natural gestures, signs, and body language to support your spoken language (see page 68).

---

## CASE STUDY: SCREAMING TO COMMUNICATE

I had a mother walk into my drop-in clinic with her 12-month-old son, named Ali, who was constantly screaming in a bloodcurdling, extremely high-pitched tone. His mother had initially thought that he was trying to communicate, but the screaming had become so persistent, upsetting, and difficult—especially when in public places or with friends or family—that she felt she couldn't cope anymore and had become worried that there was something wrong with him. She was desperate to see a professional for some specialist advice—first, to know if there was something wrong and, second, to know how to deal with the screaming.

I understood immediately what she was going through because my daughter, Jess, went through exactly the same phase. It seems to happen from around 7 to 12 months, just when your child is starting to babble and communicate intentionally, when they have a greater understanding of what's happening in his world but lack the ability to make their wants or needs understood. While there isn't an official term for it, I've seen (and heard) it so many times that I simply call it the screaming phase.

For example, if Jess saw me getting a yogurt out of the fridge in the morning for her packed lunch to take to day care, she'd scream like a banshee, which meant she wanted one now. The way I dealt with it was not to react to the scream by raising my voice but rather to respond in a quieter voice than normal so she had to shush to hear me. I would then say, "Yes, Jess wants a yoggie"—while doing the sign for yogurt, then add, "eat at Lyn's house," therefore, acknowledging and affirming her communication but not giving it to her (she would have it when she got to Lyn's house). Giving her the yogurt would have reinforced the scream as a reasonable and effective way to communicate.

I won't lie—it took a lot of patience and repetition but, in a month or two, she was using the sign for yogurt rather than screaming for it. At this age, children can get frustrated if they don't get what they want, so signing really is a life saver.

Also I tried not to ignore the screaming. Jess's screaming was a direct attempt at communication and, if I did ignore it, it would get even louder, which is not helpful.

Ali's mother was delighted to hear that a speech-language professional had also had similar issues with screaming, and she was reassured that it was perfectly normal and natural—and, in fact, a sign that Ali was potentially a very good communicator! I gave her a sheet of basic signs and never heard from her again, which I took to be a good sign—excuse the pun!

## Chapter 4

# What to do when . . . your toddler isn't attempting words

The moment a child starts saying "ma-ma" or "da-da" is a moment parents treasure forever. Generally, a child might start uttering some attempts at real words with meaning and in the right context between 12 and 14 months, and although the goo-goos and ga-gas might overlap for a bit, by the age of 18 months we hope a child will have ten to twenty real words. "Real" words can be very loose. A word to a speech therapist is any consistent vocalization for the same person or object; for example, if your little one always says "me-me" meaning meow-meow for a cat, that would be considered a word. It's so much fun to hear all the weird and wonderful words for objects or people that children use when they attempt to speak.

But what if your little one hasn't begun to say their first words? Perhaps you've already noticed that your child isn't as babbly as their pals, which might be when you first notice that there might be a delay. This is the type of child I see most regularly in my clinic. They're often between 16 and 24 months old, not speaking, and the parents are either not sure whether they should or shouldn't be worried or definitely worried and not sure how best to help. Well, without further ado, let's get started!

In the speech therapy world we use a statistic that a child needs to hear a word at least 500 times, in its context, before they will start to say it. So, hopefully you have already started being very repetitive with your language—perhaps you've been saying "up" every time you pick up your child, "car" every time a car passes, and "hello" every time they see you.

Does your child now understand a few simple words? Think very carefully about this. Does your child actually *understand* the words? They may say routine phrases—such as "Where's your shoes?" before you head out the door or "Light on" when you stand next to the light switch—without actually understanding them. Remember, your child has to understand words before they will want to use the words functionally (remember the language cake in chapter 1!).

The key to increasing understanding is using the Say What You See strategy as much as you can throughout the day and especially in your daily 10 minutes of Special Time (page 19). Persistence, patience, and praise will work wonders. The more you repeat the same words over and over again, play the same games over and over again (while not putting pressure on them to repeat your words), and reward any attempt your child makes to copy, the more progress you'll see.

You'll also have to think laterally about what your child might be saying as the words won't be completely clear when your child starts to speak. This is because they are still fine-tuning the neural pathways and practicing using their facial and mouth muscles to form the intricate movements needed to make specific sounds.

First, though, let's look at how babbling develops into gibberish.

## My little one's talking gibberish

Of course, babies don't just stop babbling and start talking. The babble begins to change over time, and children start talking gibberish, conversational babble, or, in the speech therapy world, jargon.

What does this sound like? It's as if they're telling you the most elaborate story you have ever heard, with varied tones and many different consonants. It sounds as if they are talking in a foreign language, and they look at you as if you should understand every word, whereas in actual fact you don't have the foggiest idea what they're going on about.

If you haven't already seen it, I recommend you watch the YouTube clip of the toddler twins talking to each other (search for "Talking Twin Babies")—it really is the perfect example of gibberish in action. They don't yet have any real words and aren't even using sophisticated consonants, but they're having an intricate chat using intonation, gesture, turn-taking, body language, and appropriate sentence length (see the skills on the plate of the Language Cake, page 15). It's as hilarious as it is fascinating, and you get the impression they know exactly what they are talking about.

Enjoy this slightly comical gibberish while you can, because fairly quickly, perhaps as early as 20 months, the gibberish goes away almost entirely, as children's proper attempts at words tend to take over.

Before they reach this stage, you need to encourage your child to copy the people around them as much as possible in order to get them babbling. It may sound silly, but it's a key step along the way to proper words because it enables them to practice putting a variety of consonants and vowels together in single "words" or "sentences" and experiment with elaborate intonation patterns, continuously creating those crucial neural pathways.

Alongside the gibberish, you may hear more of those long strings of babble sounds (reduplicated babble, page 51) that we encouraged in the previous chapter—"gu-gu-gu" or "ta-ta-ta"—especially incorporating the consonant sounds that your child hasn't mastered yet and which you should try to encourage if you can. There will also be some shortened utterances—listen for "uh," "ah," "ba," "ga" and so on, perhaps accompanied by pointing at a particular object or person. You will probably also hear "ah" quite often, as in "give me that," or to seek attention—for example, when your child wants to do something, like hold on to your toothbrush or climb the stairs, and knows they shouldn't.

The first consonant sounds you should hear are "m," "p," "b," followed by "d," "n," "w," "h," but again, each child is different and will do things at their own pace. Right up until 14 months, my daughter, Jess, couldn't say "d" or "n" and I was very aware of this. She said "g" instead—a sound that, developmentally, usually comes a little later. This meant "dada" was "ga-ga," which rather amused me, and water was also "ga-ga."

So don't worry too much about the sounds you are hearing at this age. Just be aware that your child should be making consonant sounds as well as vowel sounds in a meaningful way, trying to get their message across.

Want to boost your child's gibberish? Below are some Top Tip games to encourage just that. It is important to adjust the way you communicate to make it easy for your little one to understand you, so they will try to copy your words. Reduce the number of words you say to single words when drawing their attention to something, sharing a book, or playing together.

**Top Tip Time** **Copycat**

Because language development is all about being a copycat, it's very important to teach your child how to copy so they can begin to "model" (or copy) your language. Remember—everything that you do with them will be helping with the building blocks toward spoken language, and on some days, it can feel like their brain is a sponge.

The easiest way to develop your child's ability to copy is through play. In fact, you will have already been doing this with games such as peekaboo and the action songs you have been singing. Copying nonverbally in play is a prerequisite to copying verbally.

I remember running a playgroup for toddlers and one day I was playing peekaboo with Mattie and Rory when, suddenly, Amelie, who was on the other side of the room, and not really part of the game, picked up a piece of paper and started playing peekaboo, too. She was copying! This is such an important skill to learn for later language development.

There are many things you can do to encourage your child to copy you. My husband and I play Rock, Paper, Scissors to determine who will change Jess's latest dirty nappy and now Jess joins in, too, because she has learned to copy us. (Unfortunately, if she loses, she doesn't follow through with the punishment and change her own nappy!) Here are some other games to try.

- Fill two boxes with identical items, such as musical instruments and sensory objects (for example, a sponge, a dish brush, a washcloth, spoons, and a foil food wrapper). These are known as copy boxes. Give your little one a box and you keep the other. Whatever your child does, simply copy her every move. Then try role reversal.

- Sing this song from *The Tweenies*, a popular British children's television show. It goes like this.

  *Everybody do this, do this, do this. Everybody do this just like me!*

  As you sing, make an action for your child to copy— patting your knees or your lap, touching your nose, or shaking your hands. Once you've sung it through once, say, "Your turn," then copy literally anything your child is doing with their hands, and then sing again. It's great fun and very catchy!

- Encourage your child to copy you as you play. Try hugging a baby doll, banging two blocks together, bouncing a tiny ball and so on.

- Play copycat games in the mirror using noises and sounds. The key lies in waiting. You say something and wait for your child to respond before making more sounds.

- Sing familiar nursery rhymes and change the lyrics to babble noises. For example, to the tune of "Twinkle, Twinkle, Little Star," sing "da-da, da-da, da-da-da," and to the tune of "I'm a Little Teapot," sing "wa-wa, wa-wa, wa, wa"—you get the gist!

# HOW FIRST WORDS EMERGE

Alongside the gibberish, you will hear your child say the occasional real word—remember that the speech and language therapy definition of *word* is a consistently spoken utterance that represents a particular object or person. These attempts need to be repeated and praised in order for them to be heard again.

I often hear a parent say, "I think he said 'ball'!" and I say, "Yes, great! If you think he did, then he definitely did say 'ball,' and the more you repeat and praise his attempts, the more that word will appear." This is how language develops—a child almost accidentally says something and then gets lots of praise or attention, so they say it again and again.

This happened once when I was bathing Jess. I had forgotten a towel, so I called to my mother-in-law, saying, "Pat! Pat!," and no sooner had I stopped than my little parrot started shouting, "Pa! Pa!" She received a big laugh and another rendition from me, "Pat! Pat!," so she said it again and again. Great fun—although possibly not so much fun for Pat who was then at Jess's beck and call!

And this is why I love this phase—the emergence of first words. Things start to get really interesting as your child's personality begins to shine through.

**Top Tip Time** **Games for emerging words**

### Say What You See

I mentioned this technique before (in fact, hopefully, you've heard it a million times by now). Whether your bouncing baby is just a few months old or a tiny toddler, I still look upon Say What You See as *the* most important—and simple—technique a parent can use to boost their speech and communication skills.

It is so crucial to give your child a running commentary of what they are doing when they play. In other words, you must put their thought to word, as they explore and play, so that they can hear that word time and time again in its context, remember the word and begin to try to say it themselves. For example, if your child

- has a favorite game—say, stacking rings—add a repetitive commentary. In this case, you could say, "On. On. On," each time a ring is added.
- loves being chased around the sitting room, say, "Fast. Fast. Fast," or "Run. Run. Run."
- bangs their spoon on their high chair while eating, say, "Bang. Bang. Bang."
- loves watching the cars go by, say "car" every time one passes.

Remember to keep your language simple—so you would say "car" rather than "another car." You may think you sound foolish but, I assure you, you are doing the best thing for your child's language development.

Don't get into the habit of asking, "What's that? What's that?" or you might end up with a child who says "da"—"that"—for everything. Instead of asking, "What's that?," use the Say What You See technique and name objects—"tree," "dog," "bus," or "bird." This way, your child will be learning the words they need at a level that suits them.

If you feel the need to test your child to see if they know the name of an object, say, "It's a . . . ," then look at them encouragingly and pause to see if they want to fill in the gap. If they don't, say the word for them.

## Name family members

Make a scrapbook or buy a small album for photos of your little one's nearest and dearest loved ones. At this stage, only say their names—for example, Mummy, Daddy, Granddad, Baby Will, and Auntie Jo Jo (we tend to repeat the syllables, as this is closer to the kinds of utterances we are hearing from your little babbler).

You could even try making a PowerPoint presentation or on-line album of family members so that your child can flip through the pictures on an iPad.

## ONE WORD FITS ALL: OVEREXTENSION

Sometimes early talkers tend to use the same word to refer to a number of different objects. This is known as overextension. So, for example, "wawa" may refer to any liquid, even if it's not actually water, and "car" might refer to literally anything that moves! You will also soon discover that children usually repeat the first syllable in a word, so two-syllable words will most probably be spoken as a repetition of the same syllable (for instance, mama, dada, and baba). For example, my nephew used to say, "More more car car" when referring to watching a train clip on YouTube until he was about 3 years old. This means that you'll find yourself translating your child's language for those who don't know it very well and aren't used to their quirky speech. Don't worry about this. It's perfectly normal and will soon pass once your child realizes there is a clearer way to get their message across. Just continue to praise their attempts at language and model the correct word—"Yes, train. You want to watch more trains." (Read more on modeling words, page 82.) It's also possible for children to underuse words. This is known as underextension (see page 178).

### Have a word theme for the day

Collect objects that relate to a specific word and play with them for the day, for instance. Peppa Pig, doggy, dinosaur, etc. (You should also learn the sign for the word so that your child is bombarded with it through their eyes and ears.) The objects you collect might include a book, an item of clothing, a bag, and a toy, and you could even sing a familiar song. Let me expand on this using the words "bear" and "up." You could

- read a book about a bear,
- have a teddy bears' picnic and encourage your child to give some food and drink to the bears,
- sing "We're Going on a Bear Hunt,"

- bring a bear to lunch with you or take them for a walk with you—put him on the swings, too,
- throw bears in a box and say, "Bye-bye, bear," then bring them out one by one and say, "Hello, bear,"
- look up bears on Google Images and say "bear" every time you see one, and/or
- let your child wear their bear pajamas for the day.

You can use this format for any object you think your little one is interested in, and if you can't think of a song that fits your theme, simply change the words to a familiar song.

### Going UP!!!

Another good word to focus on at this stage is *up* because it's a high-frequency word that is easy to say. Think how many times you can say "up" in a day—lift up, get up, pick up, build up, go up, tidy up, clean up, mop up, up in the sky, upside down, up to Mummy . . . the list is endless.

You could cut out pictures from a catalog with things that depict up and down—such as fire engines with ladders on top, dollhouses with stairs, garages with steps, slides, toy umbrellas, and sandcastles and stick them into a scrapbook. Other ideas include singing "Itsy Bitsy Spider" (climbing "up" the waterspout), "Jack and Jill" (went "up" the hill), and "Roly Poly, Roly Poly, Up Up Up" (self-explanatory). Also, repeat saying "up" while sucking through a straw or blowing up a balloon.

### Try playing What's in the Bag?

Put objects within a category into a bag and play What's in the Bag? Give the bag a shake to generate a bit of enthusiasm in the game, then say, "What's in the bag?" and encourage your child to pull something out of it. I usually sing a song to the tune of "Old MacDonald Had a Farm" that goes like this.

> *What's in the bag?*
> *What's in the bag?*
> *E-I-E-I-O*

Then either you or your child should pull out an object and you say, "It's a . . . [wait to give your child a chance to say a sound but, if they don't, complete the sentence] . . . car."

Make different sets of similar types of objects, such as some balls, a set of hats or a handful of spoons. This way, your baby can copy you and, hopefully, as the bag empties out and you repeat "ball" each time you bring one out, they will attempt to say the word when you say, "It's a . . . ?," looking at them encouragingly.

Alternatively, try a small range of objects that fit within a certain category or set—for example, vehicles, clothes, snacks, toys, or animals. Interestingly, when words are learned within their particular sets, they are stored better in the language center in the brain (a bit like a filing cabinet in your brain). This then makes it easier for a child to retrieve them in order to say the words when they are needed.

Name each item as you pull it out and then throw it into a large container—children at this age love "container play" and it's a technique I use all the time at my clinic. Continue until the bag is empty and then enthusiastically start all over again.

**Top Tip Time** **Giving your child reasons to communicate**

Let's face it, we all need a little encouragement at times—and I am a firm believer in the power of dangling that metaphorical carrot. Your child won't necessarily talk unless they are motivated to do so and you'd be amazed at how easy it is to entice them into communicating with you when they want to get their little hands on something. Lots of opportunities to do this will naturally crop up during the day. Here are some examples.

**Offer choices**

When your child is reaching or pointing, even when you know what they want, offer a choice. So, if they reach for a banana, you pick up a banana and a plate and say, "Banana or plate?" This gives them the model of the words you want them to say, and if you hold the objects on either side of your face, they can look at your mouth to see how it moves to form the word.

### "Ask an adult" games

These are toys or games that require an adult to activate and can be used in conjunction with the infinitely useful word *more*. (Once your child has mastered it, they can use "more" to communicate their desire for anything from water to cheese to tickling.) So, if your child wants more toy action, they will have a reason to communicate with you.

Objects that require adult input include balloons, bubbles, spinning tops and wind-up musical toys. Show your child how the game works. For example, run the car down the track or blow up a balloon and let it go, then encourage your child to ask for "more."

I always use the sign, too. If you are just beginning to use signs, try hand-over-hand signing, which means you mold your little one's hand into the shape of the sign. I started this when Jess was 12 months old and it took just 10 minutes for her to pick up that she had to move her hands together to get some "more" bubbles—I was amazed.

Try playing with a toy that requires your child to ask for pieces so it will work—for example, a tower made of blocks, a train track or a puzzle. Hold the pieces back and encourage them to ask for "more." You can also do this with food—give your child a very small piece of cookie instead of the whole thing and encourage them to ask for "more."

### Asking for help

You can try putting your child's favorite toy or food in a see-through container or bag so that they have to ask you to get it out for them. This works for puzzles, too, where an adult is needed to help put the piece in. Encourage your child to sign or say, "Help me" or "Open."

### Sharing books

The new way of saying "read a book" is "share a book," which I like because it suggests that your child is taking an active part in the process. So, encourage them to do this right from infancy by offering them a choice, such as "Do you want a bear book or a tickle book?" and wait for them to point or attempt to say "bear" or "tickle."

When sharing the book, keep your language simple—you don't have to follow the text, just say single words or short phrases of a level that is right for your child. At my clinic I usually simplify and personalize the book (by using the child's finger to point to the things I know they are interested in) and then, every so often, I read the book as it is written—especially when it has a rhyme or a rhythm—which will help with later speech-sound development and will extend concentration span.

When reading, say the word (for example, "cow") and encourage your child to copy you by looking at them expectantly or saying, "It's a . . ." and pausing to allow them to try to finish the sentence (only finishing it yourself if they don't). You can try a role reversal, where you point to a picture and look at them expectantly to see if they say something.

Use books that have the same pictures on every page or in a repetitive line so that your child can join in (for example, *Dear Zoo* by Rod Campbell).

### Is your baby attempting first words?

It takes some parents a while to realize that when their child attempts a word like "bye-bye," their initial attempt might sound more like "dye-dye" but if you watch and think laterally you can notice their attempt and reward their effort. And this attempt at the word needs to be rewarded or your child won't know to try and say it again.

"Hiya" is another example. A lot of children might start saying, "Hiya!" and you think to yourself, "I never say 'hiya,' I always say 'hello.'" Well, "hiya" is a very immature way of saying "hello" and as the parent recognizes "hiya" and models "hiya" rather than "hello," the child enjoys saying and repeating the word over and over again.

As you know, a word is defined as a consistent utterance in response to the same stimulus, so listen for consistent sounds or responses each time your little one sees the same object or action.

Having watched children say their first words for many years now, I've noticed that most attempt the same words in the same way—you might hear "bo-bo" for "bottle," "mmm" for "more," "ga-ga" for "daddy," or "dar" for "car." But to an untrained ear these are not obvious words. I've had some parents come to see me to say that their child isn't talking and I've immediately been able to "translate" their words for the parents, who were delighted to realize that speech was, in fact, well on its way but not clear to the untrained ear just yet.

So, just to reiterate, don't be disappointed if you can't recognize the actual word your child is trying to say; just listen for any consistent sound or noise for a particular object or action and establish what they are using the word to refer to. Once you have cracked this you can keep repeating the word back ("Yes, that's right, it's a CAR!") and they will soon learn the clarity of the word perfectly.

Use Say What You See, repeat words, simplify your language, keep your language consistent, and stick to what your child is familiar with (always using the same phrase for a specific activity or item; for example, say "Let's eat!" at each mealtime rather than "It's din-dins," "Snack time!," or countless other variables). Your child will start to attempt to copy things you do and say. And you will be rewarded with lots of lovely words!

Often, there can be a lot of frustration during this phase and sometimes screams can be heard rather than first word attempts (see earlier case study, page 77). You might encounter this scenario if your child is given one grape instead of the whole bunch, if another child comes near their toy, or if something falls on the floor. Try to stay calm and say the words that describe what has happened or what the child wants—"More grapes, Mummy," "Lou Lou's turn," "Book gone," and so on.

While being calm and patient will help, I have already mentioned that the very best way to minimize your child's frustration is to give them another form of communication—signing.

### Top Tip Time  Attempting first words

Help your child make that first leap from experimental noises into words by trying the Top Tip games below. In these games, you repeat the same words over and over again during everyday routines so you create a habit of saying a particular word in a particular instance. Here are some examples.

- Line up some toys by the bath and say, "Ready, set, splash!" as they fall into the water. Then, once your child is familiar with this habit, say, "Ready, set . . ." and wait to see if they attempt the word. Whatever they say, give them lots of praise, because this might be an attempt at the real word and, over time, it'll begin to sound more and more like it.

- Use the same technique for, "Wash, wash, wash. Wash, wash . . ." as you wash their body, and "Rub, rub, rub. Rub, rub . . ." as you dry them with a towel.

- Your little one will love climbing up the stairs, so climb with them and say, "Up, up, up." They may first say "buh" or "uh" so reward these attempts.

- "Diddle diddle" can be an early attempt at "tickle tickle," so say, "One, two, three, tickle. One, two, three . . ." whenever you tickle them.

- Say, "Ready, set . . . go!," then chase your child around the room.

- Say, "Clothes off!" when you are getting them ready for bed. Get specific . . . "Sock off, sock off, pants off, top off," and so on.

- If your child is really enjoying something, encourage them to say, "More," and make the sign for "more," too—this works especially well at mealtimes, when they'll be rewarded with another spoonful.
- Laugh when other people around you are laughing and encourage them to join in. Look at them and say, "Ha ha ha."
- Say, "Bye-bye," during container play each time you put a block into the box.
- Say, "Wheee," when a dolly or your child goes down the slide.
- Try reading a book with a repetitive line, such as "Brown bear brown . . . ," and see if your child can complete the last word.

Whether your child's first word is *cake* or *cat* (or "buh-gah," in the case of my daughter, Jess), many children attempt their first real words at around 12 to 18 months. And once they start seeing the impact of delivering a "real" word, things begin to get really exciting because children begin to pick up more and more and their personality shines through.

When your child hits the magic 50-word mark, they tend to try to copy everything, instigating a language explosion. Until this point, though, they might have picked up a word here and there, with no real speed or urgency, which will leave you champing at the bit for more. This is totally normal, so just enjoy the words they do have and trust that more are on the way.

You'll recognize some of the skills I cover in this chapter from previous sections—expanding your child's language, understanding, listening, and social skills. But now I'll show you how to take them up a notch, making the games and interactive play slightly more complex so that you stay that one crucial developmental step ahead of your little one, effortlessly encouraging them on to the next stage.

# KEEPING ONE STEP AHEAD OF YOUR CHILD'S UNDERSTANDING

As I've mentioned before, don't forget how important your child's level of understanding is. You have to keep *your* language level one step ahead of your little one's so that you can help them soak up all the words you say. A child needs to understand words before they attempt to say them and, for an SLP, a child's understanding is far more important than their ability to express themself at this age, as it is a better indication of their intelligence level.

In order to understand something, you have to listen to, process, and remember words and, as you can imagine, every day, this sequence is happening over and over again. Typically a child at 12 months, might understand between 3 and 50 words. By 18 months they could be capable of understanding at least 50 words.

## INSTINCTIVELY SIMPLIFYING LANGUAGE— FROM "GAAA" TO "WATER"

Deb Roy, director of the Center for Communication at the Massachusetts Institute of Technology, wanted to understand how his infant son learned language. So, in 2005 he wired up his house with video cameras to catch every moment (with exceptions!) of his son's life, then studied 90,000 hours of home video to watch his utterance of "gaaa" slowly turn into "water." The Human Speechome Project is the largest-ever study of child language development in a natural or clinical environment.[1]

By collecting each instance in which his son heard a word and noting the context, Roy and his team mapped all 530 words the boy learned by his second birthday. In doing so, they uncovered a surprising pattern, which was that caregivers used simpler language the closer the boy got to grasping a word. At the point they sensed he was on the cusp of getting it, all three primary caregivers—Roy, his wife, and their nanny—simplified their language to guide him to the word, then gently guided him toward more complex language once he had grasped it.

Roy says, "We were all systematically, and I would think subconsciously, restructuring our language to meet him at the moment of the birth of the word and then bringing him gently into more complex language."

Roy says this provides evidence that caregivers modify their language at a level never reported or suspected before. It's not just that his son was learning from his linguistic environment; "the environment was learning from him," says Roy. (Perform a Google search for "Deb Roy: The Birth of a Word" to watch Roy's fascinating talk on his findings.)

But how do you know what your child understands? I remember going to see a speech therapy friend of mine some years ago whose daughter was quite little. She said, "I know I shouldn't really do this, but watch this . . ." SLPs frown upon parents who continuously quiz and question their children, but she sat her daughter down with a range of objects spread out in front of her and said, "Where's the owl/squirrel/frog?" Her daughter knew all of these and more—an extensive range of fairly abstract animals—and I was amazed. So, from time to time, try something like this—"Where's the . . . ?," "What does a . . . say?," or "Where's your . . . ?" (see the following Top Tip Time games).

Just remember to be careful with questions. You don't want your little one to feel that they are continuously being tested. If you overdo it, they won't want to play or talk with you so much. Pick your moment carefully. Remember that, ultimately, you need to be there for your child as their language model and not their examiner!

**Top Tip Time** **Promoting good understanding of language**

### Keep it consistent

I want to reiterate the importance of sticking to the same standard words and phrases. In English, there are so many ways to say the same thing—"Bedtime," "Time for a little sleep," "Let's go bye-byes," "Off to bed," and so on. If you can, use just one of these phrases consistently so your little one can understand and anticipate what you are going to say, and try to copy you.

Once you feel you are regularly using the same words and phrases during your daily routine, trigger your child into talking by starting a well-used phrase (a carrier phrase), thereby encouraging the missing word to just pop out. When you start the phrase, look at them questioningly and leave a gap for them to fill in the last word. If they don't, do it for them (for example, "It's time for ... lunch," "Open the ... door," "Ready, set ... go," and "Drink your ... milk").

### Where's the ... ?/Where's your ... ? games

Be selective about the objects you ask your child to point to and think of the key words in their environment. Say, "Where's the light/door/window/nose/hair/eyes/cat/dog/cookie?" and encourage them to point. If they don't respond, point at the objects for them and say the word at the same time. Remember to give lots of praise if they get it right and, if they get it wrong, praise their effort.

Home in on one word and repeat it over and over again. For example, in the bath, it is also fun to encourage your child to wash different parts of their body in the bath with lots of bubbles or in the sitting room, hide favorite objects in fairly obvious places and encourage your child to find them.

## Matching object to object

Assemble pairs of balls, shoes, socks, spoons, cars, teddies, nappies, bananas, and so on. Mix them up and see if your child can find the "same." If they can manage this, try object-to-picture matching, which is slightly harder. Lay two pictures on the floor, one matching the object you have chosen and one of a different object. Say, "Find the same," and encourage your child to put the object on its correlating picture.

## Say What You See

Remember to use the Say What You See technique when you are playing or are out and about. Look at what your child is looking at and model the words they need, so they can try to say them for themselves next time they see the same objects.

## HOW THE BRAIN STORES WORDS

In the language center in your brain there's a metaphorical area called the semantic center, which is where all your words are processed and stored. In 1997, professors Joy Stackhouse and Bill Wells of Sheffield University came up with a Speech Processing Model that explains this process.[2] They mapped the chain of events that occurs when a new word is heard, recognized as being English, decoded into the sounds that it's made up of, and understood. Their findings suggest that a word is stored in a very organized way, so it can be retrieved as easily as possible when the person wants to say that word. This means that the brain cleverly splits up words and stores them in categories. Below is a list of the categories in which words are stored in the brain, according to Stackhouse and Wells.

- By their meaning: farm animals, clothes, body parts and so on
- Words with the same sounds at the beginning or end, like "pan," "peg," "poor," "pig," or "map," "up," "cup," "shop"

- Words with the same syllable structure: for example, "elephant," "strawberry," "telephone" or "television," "avocado," "caterpillar"

- Words that rhyme: for instance, "cat" and "mat"

- Words with the same vowel: for example, "kite," "my," and "night"

If only my paper-filing system were this robust!

## WHAT TO DO IF YOUR CHILD ISN'T VERY SOCIABLE

### Being sociable with you

At around 12 to 18 months, your child should become more and more sociable. They usually begin to take notice of more things going on around them, pointing to things that interest them, like photos on the wall. They are finding innovative ways to get your attention, like yanking your hair, throwing food on the floor, or clinging to your leg. And they will pass objects to you or strangers to see what responses they get.

You should notice your little one starting to imitate the things you do, like pretending to brush their hair or drinking from a mug that you've just put down. They are noticing what is happening, retaining the information, and copying it. This then helps them to learn that there is a sequence to events which, later, develops into forming a sequence of words into a sentence or a sequence of events into a story. As they use these objects in play and practice turn-taking with them, the skills they pick up will transfer to turn-taking in a conversation.

Children tend to enjoy being center stage and think the world revolves around them. They are entirely egocentric. They might join in when people around them are laughing—having no idea what the joke is—and enjoy trying to make you laugh, too. You'll see them peeping through their legs when they're standing up, clapping when you clap, making a funny noise, hand-jiving or bopping their bodies up and down to music—all to get a giggle from their adoring audience. They simply love attention and applause. All this encourages them to become more and more socially interactive. The more input they get from their closest adults the more they learn more from them.

## How to encourage being sociable with peers

Your child may take notice of others by pulling their hair, chasing after them, handing them things, or snatching things from them. They are becoming curious about other children, but at this stage they don't really "play" together.

Children usually begin playing in parallel with other children at around 18 months, which means they'll play the same game next to each other rather than play the same game together—imagine two children playing in parallel at a sandbox.

## How to encourage pretend play

Pretend play means putting a phone to their ear, pretending to brush their teeth, eating a toy banana, or even pretending to go to sleep (especially when singing "Rock-a-Bye Baby," in my experience!).

Researchers suggest that there are clear links between pretend play and social and linguistic competence. This is because pretense encourages the young child to use their imagination and memory for situations and experiences and to use language for thinking things through. They are thinking of a familiar scenario in their head, then acting it out. This process can also help concentration, problem solving, and reasoning.

See how the process evolves using a spoon. At first, a baby might bang a spoon. The next time, they might pretend they're eating. Then they might try to feed a toy doll. They could then go on to pretend to use the spoon to cook, or at a higher level of play skills, to use a spoon in an imaginative way such as symbolizing it as a seesaw!

First, encourage your baby to feed you or help you drink at mealtimes. Then take a cup, bowl, and spoon and take turns giving each other a drink. Make a big slurping noise so it's very dramatic and entertaining for your child. Now take turns feeding each other.

Your child may look completely bewildered—this is normal, just carry on. Once they start enjoying it, they will be inclined to join in.

Next, take a doll and a teddy and encourage your child to become part of the game. You could go through the bath, bedtime story, and bed routine with the dolly. Take teddy with you on outings and include him as part of the family. Your aim is to encourage two-step sequences and then more—for example, bathe teddy, dry him, then put on his pajamas.

**Top Tip Time** **The power of play**

### Making friends

First, arrange to meet up on a regular basis with parents of two or three other children. Fun outings at this age include trips to hands-on children's museums, playgrounds, petting zoos, or anywhere that children can run around freely. (Just remember that at first your child is more likely to engage in parallel play than to play cooperatively with their friends.)

Point out other children in your child's environment and talk to your child about what those children are doing. Encourage your child to first watch the other children and then to either copy their play, play a simple turn-taking game with them, or just play alongside.

Remember—at this age you should encourage your child to interact with a wide range of people of all ages, in different environments.

# TESTING YOUR TOLERANCE— TEMPER TANTRUMS

It's common for a child to start testing their parents' boundaries around the age of 2 or even older if your child has a delay. This may include deliberately throwing or dropping toys or food on the floor, refusing to be strapped into the car seat, and continuously trying to alter their parents' plans through persuasion and protest—"Noooooo."

Why is this? We say that all behavior is communication, meaning that by having a tantrum, your child is trying to tell you something. All children go through a phase like this. They might be trying to tell you that they want to become more independent, that they want to accomplish a new task, or to be able to communicate on their own, but they don't yet have the necessary skills to succeed. It can therefore be a very frustrating time for them and having a tantrum is their way of expressing this.

Distract your child in such situations. Try to predict or preempt a tantrum by keeping a close eye out—if they have trouble putting a shape into a shape sorter, or putting their shorts on independently, give them a helping hand. Tantrums are more likely to occur when a child is tired or hungry, so if you're going somewhere important, give your child an early nap and an early lunch.

I remember driving Jess around the neighborhood before her third birthday party so she'd have a quick nap and, being more rested, hopefully not have an outburst at her party. We had a minor tantrum over putting Hula-Hoops chips on each finger without their breaking, but she was certainly easier to manage than she would have been without that snooze in the car!

## EMOTIONAL DEVELOPMENT

When your child cries and gets angry and frustrated, help them to understand their emotions by voicing them out loud. For example, you could say, "You're sad because Daddy's gone to work," or "You're angry because there are no more cookies."

Children usually love it when a parent does this; they feel better understood with regard to their feelings and will hopefully be happier and more content accordingly.

## Try to use TV time constructively

There is a lot of evidence that if the TV is on all the time in a home as background noise, it will reduce the number of conversations held, and that can hinder language development during this crucial 0-to-48-month period. For this reason, many experts recommend that children under the age of 2 not watch any TV at all.

But I am a realist and I know that TV time is sometimes a lifesaver—as when you're able to pop your little one in front of the TV for 5 minutes while you unload the dishwasher or fold the laundry. The good news is that you can use TV constructively. Here's how.

If your child is watching TV, ensure it is a program for children. It may seem as if I am stating the obvious, but you'd be surprised. A lot of research goes into children's shows these days, with psychologists and language experts all consulted to create a program that is eye-catching and informative.

To get the most out of a program, your child needs to engage with it—so the TV isn't just a background noise, it is the activity. This means that, ideally, you should be sitting right beside your child, pointing things out, making comments, repeating catchphrases, and making links with your own life. So, if the program is showing a teddy bears' picnic, encourage your child to gather her teddies, too. Once the program is over, act out what you have just seen. For example, if it was about a postal worker, get out a toy car and pretend you are delivering the mail.

If you are doing chores while your child is watching TV, you can still follow this advice, just to a lesser extent. So, if you are tidying up and see that it's raining in *Thomas the Tank Engine* world, you can say, "Oh, look, it's raining in our backyard, too."

Personally, I also find that TV can be useful as part of a routine. For example, Jess always had a bath at 6:00 PM and then we'd sit on the sofa together and watch an episode of one of her favorite bedtime shows, followed by a couple of books before her bedtime. This became such a well-established routine that I'd worry when we'd go away!

I am not going to give you a guideline of how many minutes of TV a day are acceptable—I realize that every day is different. The crucial thing to remember is that you shouldn't use the TV as company for your child and that even though children's programs are well made these days, they're never going to be as good as you! You are always the best resource for educational achievement and good language development that your child has. Don't have the TV on constantly and be strict about switching it off once you move on to a new activity.

Having said all that, there is one thing I am militant about when it comes to TV, and that is to never have the TV on during mealtimes. Many of my work families and friends have fallen into a pattern of doing this, arguing that a program will distract their child so that they will mindlessly spoon food into their mouth and end up eating more—without turning the dinner table into a battleground. I am very against this.

Eating should be the most sociable time of the day; you are facing each other, so your child can watch your mouth as you talk, and it's the perfect opportunity for the whole family to chat with each other. Even if you have the TV on in the morning while you go about your routine, you should always turn it off before breakfast. The same goes for lunch and dinner. I know that weaning can be tricky and that most children are fussy when it comes to food but TV is not the answer, so please turn it off at mealtimes.

## Overly enthusiastic nodding and head shaking

Some babies seem to start nodding and/or shaking their heads at around 6 to 8 months, but others, much later. Once they've picked it up, some seem to do it to excess, becoming little head bangers who wouldn't look out of place in the front row of a heavy metal concert. They nod or shake for "yes" or "no," when they are excited, when they are tired, and at almost any opportunity they get.

Parents can see this as a cause for concern (there are forums full of worried posts from parents on this matter on the internet), but it's all perfectly normal and a natural stage (I've even heard one pediatrician say that it may be because they enjoy the sensation of feeling slightly dizzy!). Remember when your baby first learned to clap and how they did it all the time? As with nodding and head shaking, once young children discover a new trick, they like to repeat it—a lot—especially when you are probably encouraging them by laughing or nodding and head shaking back.

### THE EVOLUTION OF THE HEAD SHAKE

Research indicates that the head shake, usually meaning "no," may be an inborn action and evolutionary biologists believe that it's the first gesture humans learn. This theory maintains that when the newborn baby has had enough milk, they shake their head from side to side to reject their mother's breast. Similarly, a child who has had enough to eat uses the head shake to reject attempts to spoon-feed them.

## Being careful with questions

Some parents are so desperate to know what their child knows that they get into a habit of asking too many questions. Can you hear yourself saying, "What's that?," "Where's it going?," "What color is it?," "How many teddies?" DON'T. When you ask other adults a question, they answer. When you ask children a question, they often feel under pressure, which feels unpleasant, so they back off. If someone you met continually asked you questions, you'd soon find someone else who is easier to communicate with.

I notice this a lot with children who have a language delay. They can become very reluctant to speak because their parents have put too much pressure on them to talk and as a result they tend to refuse. So, take the pressure off your child to communicate and you will find that they talk more. Instead of constantly asking questions, keep on using the Say What You See technique.

## My child makes mistakes when attempting words

When a child points to something and makes a sound, they are trying to say the word. Praise their attempt and model the correct word back—for example, "Uh—yes, a bird."

Leaving off the final consonant from a word (for example, "buh" for "bus") is perfectly normal when a child starts to speak, so praise your child's attempt and model the correct word back— "Yes, it's a 'busssss'" (you can emphasize the sound they missed).

Using an incorrect consonant at the start of a word is also very common (for instance, "duh" for "stuck"). You guessed it—praise your child's attempt and model the correct word back.

In a nutshell, you should be praising any attempt to communicate, whether it's a sign, a gesture, or a word, and modeling the correct version back in a positive way. This will help your child to want to say the word again.

## Again, again!

Children tend to like the same games and activities over and over again. It is possible that again or "aguh" might be one of your child's first attempts at a real word. There might be times that you wished the word never existed, like when you've read the same book a hundred times, and other times when you sparkle with delight, like when your little one shouts "aguh" as loudly as they can after singing their favorite song in the local music group.

Within reason, try to honor your child's request and do the same task again and again. It will really help to create those pathways that link the ear to the brain's language center, and the brain's language center to the mouth. The more your child hears the same words and phrases, the more they will understand and the more they will speak. So, say it again, Sam!

---

### CASE STUDY: WHEN THERE ARE NO WORD ATTEMPTS AT 18 MONTHS

This story is from a mother who came into my clinic.

"I'm worried about my 18-month-old son, who isn't talking at all. He was an early walker and is constantly on the move, running around everywhere. He loves to read books with me but mainly just turns the pages and lifts the flaps. He has great fun lining up cars and building towers but doesn't talk when he plays. My husband and I talk to our son constantly about what we're doing, pointing things out in the hope of encouraging him to say words, but he hardly even attempts to speak, apart from a bit of 'da-da-da-da' now and then. He definitely understands what things mean, though. If I say, 'Where's Dadda?,' he instantly runs to the door thinking Daddy is home from work. If I say 'fish,' he looks at the fish tank, but apart from saying 'boos' once or twice when asked to say 'fish,' he just isn't interested. My heart sank yesterday when I saw a little girl who couldn't have been any older than he is talking to her mum in three- to four-word sentences! He seems happy enough and is completely scrumptious. Should I be worried?"

My response to this mother, which also applies to any parent who has concerns about their child's language, is that children develop at different rates, so try not to panic prematurely. More than likely your child will be a little chatterbox before you know it. It is so important that your child *understands* language, and once they have that good understanding, their words will follow. It would be more worrying if you felt he didn't understand you.

However, there are things you can do to improve the situation.

- First of all, check your child's hearing. Go to your pediatrician and ask for your child's hearing to be evaluated.

- Use the Say What You See technique. Put your child's thoughts into words as they play at a single-word level—for example, "Ball—it's a ball. Ball." Lower your language level to single words or short phrases, repeat the key words over and over again, and start signing.

- Follow your child's interests in play and talk about the things that they are interested in. Find their motivators—be it cars, cats, or cranes!

- Have Special Time every day, when you play together and you model the language that they might be motivated to say.

- Make lots of symbolic noises as you play (for example, vehicle noises, animal noises, etc.) and add random noises like "wee" as a car goes down a ramp or "ah" when teddy is touched. These noises tend to be easier to say. Copy your child's noises and sounds, too, particularly babble sounds (for example, for dog, "wuh-wuh-wuh"; for cow, "moo-moo-moo"; and for sheep, "ba-ba-ba"), creating good pathways between the brain and the articulators. There's a great song to sing to the first line of the tune of "She'll Be Coming Round the Mountain" (you'll need a toy car, airplane, motorcycle, and train). Leave a pause for your child to fill in the noise.

*I am driving in my little motor car*—brum-brum-brum.
*I am flying in my little airplane*—zzz-zzz-zzz.
*I am riding in my great big choo choo train*—choo-choo-choo.

*I am driving on my great big motorcycle—vrum-vrum-vrum.*

- Make a babble bag and a sound sack.

- Think laterally about what they might be trying to say (for instance, "bah" instead of "ball" or "wawa" for "flower"). Through no fault of your own, you might be missing some of their attempts and then not rewarding them with a repetition or some praise.

- Don't worry about the clarity of your child's words at this point—accept all attempts, no matter how far removed from the target word. I can't tell you how many times a parent tells me a child is saying nothing, but when I visit, I see the child attempting so many words that the parent isn't catching on to.

- If it's difficult to pin your little one down to concentrate and listen to language, do more listening activities (see my suggestions on page 60–63) to help your child's ability to focus. Remember—good listening leads to good understanding, and once a child can understand, they will begin to try to talk.

- Try not to question your child all the time, however tempting this might be. It is better that you say the word so they can hear, remember, and understand it.

- If your child has a dummy, get rid of it and try to limit its use.

The range of what is considered to be "normal" (there I go with my quotes again, because I really do want you to take this word with a big pinch of salt!) during this phase of language development is massive, which is why the differences between children can seem stark to worried parents. At the top end, you might expect a boom of words and have a child who is saying two- or even three-word sentences at 24 months, but at the other end of the scale, children with only 50 single words at 24 months are considered to have perfectly normal language development, too. If this is the case, you might have to wait a little longer and keep implementing your Special Time games for their language explosion to arrive. So, without further ado, let's continue on . . .

# Chapter 5

# What to do when . . . your child only has a few words

In this chapter, I'll show you how to broaden your child's experiences and model masses of sounds, words, and phrases in order to bring on a language explosion. We'll think about the *types* of words they are using—such as family names, social words, and verbs—and I'll explain how, once they have a collection of about 50 words (covering as many of the different categories of words as possible), they'll start to join two words together—for instance, "No yoggie," "Bye Stu," or "Monkey eating." So that's where we'll begin—tips and games for expanding single words in preparation for two-word phrases.

Many 2-year-olds have a vocabulary of 75 to 225 words, but if your child has 50 words or fewer, they would be considered a late talker. If that's the case, you'll need to go back though the previous chapters in this book to find the stage your child is at— and stuck in— and put in the groundwork for the emergence of a boom in single words. Professor Leslie Rescorla, director of the Child Study Institute at Bryn Mawr College in Pennsylvania, reported that the most popular 25 words spoken by 2-year-olds are Mummy, Daddy, baby, milk, juice, hello, ball, yes, no, dog, cat, nose, eye, banana, cookie, car, hot, thank you, bath, shoe, hat, book, all gone, more, and bye-bye.[1] In the UK, Ann Locke has produced her list of the first 100 words. Words marked with an asterisk have been adapted for American English speakers.

## Nouns

| | | |
|---|---|---|
| Baby | Ball | Apple |
| Daddy | Bike | Cookie* |
| Man | Bricks | Dinner |
| Mommy* | Bus | Plate |
| Eyes | Car | Spoon |
| Feet | Doll | Sweets |
| Hair | Duck | Cup |
| Hands | Carriage/ | Drink |
| Mouth | Stroller* | Milk |
| Nose | Swing | Orange/juice |
| Toes | Teddy/Bear | Water |
| Tummy | Book | Bed |
| Bag | Box | Chair |
| Coat | Paper | House |
| Dress | Pencil | Table |
| Hat | Bird | Brush |
| Underwear* | Cat | Soap |
| Shoes | Dog | Sink* |
| Socks | Flower | Towel |
| Pants* | Tree | |

## Verbs

| | | |
|---|---|---|
| Brush | Eat | Look (at) |
| Clap | Find | Make |
| Come | Get | Play |
| Cook | Give | Push |
| Cry | Hit | Put |
| Cut | Jump | Read |
| Drink | Kick | Run |
| Dry | Like/love | Sit |

### Verbs (cont.)

| | |
|---|---|
| Sleep | Walk |
| Stand | Want |
| Throw | Wash |

### Other words

| | | |
|---|---|---|
| Big | Hot | On |
| Dirty | In | Up |
| Down | More | Wet |
| Gone | No | Yes |

Initially, your child might learn the names for their own belongings—take "shoes," for example. They will know their own shoes as "shoes" and then will learn that yours are also called shoes. They will then spot shoes on TV or in a book and realize that even though they may be different colors, shapes, and sizes, they, too, are called shoes. It's a very intricate process—first, you have to familiarize your child with the object, then help them understand its name, and then, finally, encourage them to say it. You cannot expect your child to say the word until the first two stages are complete.

Below are some activities to help your little one expand the number of single words they use.

**Top Tip Time** **Boom boosters!**

### Staying one step ahead

As you know, always try to stay one step ahead of your child's language. I heard a lovely story recently. Hugh knew that his son Oliver said "dog" for every four-legged animal he saw and "duck" for every bird, as he couldn't name any others. So, thinking that he was making it easier for his son to understand the world around him, Hugh followed suit. It wasn't until Oliver's mum heard her husband pointing out "dog, dog, dog" when they saw lambs in a field and asked, "Why are you saying dog when there are no dogs in that field?"

Hugh explained that because these were the only animals Oliver knew, he didn't want to confuse him by stirring more into the mix. But how could Oliver's language ever expand if he didn't ever hear the correct name for each animal? By talking at the same level as Oliver, Hugh wasn't extending his understanding at all. If you want your child's language to expand, you have to provide a language model at the right level—only saying "dog" and "duck" was too low a level for Oliver and therefore wouldn't encourage him to move on.

In order for a child's language to expand, you need to model the words over and over again before you can expect the child to say them. By now you should know that a better way to expand Oliver's language and extend his vocabulary would be to use the Say What You See technique—so, label all the animals, and then, once your child is able to say them, copy and add a word each time, so "duck's swimming," "Gruffalo's looking," and so on.

## TRY LEARNING NEW WORDS IN THEIR CATEGORY

Children find it easier to store words and retrieve from the language center in their brain if they learn them in their "category."

Below is a list of the categories of words you can focus on with your child. Choose a different category each week and, within that category, find all the objects you have around the house within that category—for example, books, items of clothing, or toys to play with. You could make flash cards and put them in a big box so that every day you can do your Special Time to focus on a particular category of words.

| | | |
|---|---|---|
| Family and friends | Classroom | Numbers 10 to 20 |
| Body parts | Furniture | Prepositions: in, on, under, in front, behind, next to, between. |
| Farm animals | Garden | |
| Zoo animals | Kitchen | |
| Pets | Bathroom | |
| Garden/ woodland animals | Weather | |
| | Park | |
| Food and drink | Simple verbs | Days of the week |
| | Colors | |
| Transporta- tion | Shapes | Calendar events (birthday, holidays) |
| | Numbers 1 to 10 | |
| Clothes | | |

## Mailing games

Make up a few sets of flash cards using pictures from catalogs or Google Images stuck onto cardboard; perhaps laminate them, and keep them in your Special Time Box. Make sets using the category themes above.

Encourage your child to name them—for instance, "It's a . . . bed"—before they put them into an old shoebox. They'll love it.

## Other flash card games

Get hold of a simple pack of flash cards—they can be useful in lots of word games, such as in the following ideas.

- **Bowling:** Stand your flash cards up against plastic bowling pins (or old toilet-paper rolls) and take turns instructing each other on which picture to knock down.
- **Stepping stones:** Lay the cards on the floor and tell each other which picture to jump on.
- **Clothesline:** Hang your pictures on a clothesline with your child; this will help develop fine motor skills, too. Just string a line between a couple of chairs.

- **Hunt the picture:** Hide the pictures around your room and hunt them down. Find them and then say what they are.
- **Fishing game:** Find a magnet and tie it onto a string. Put a paper clip on each picture. Now fish for the cards and then name them.
- **Memory games:** Show two of the cards to your child, put them facedown on the table in front of you and say, "Where's the cow?," "Where's the pig?" Then extend the number of cards your child has to remember to three. Another idea is to find objects that fit within a particular category and match one object to another, then an object to a picture. You could do this using a plastic milk carton cut in half—stick the picture of an object on the outside and then get your child to place the real object inside the milk carton. When they have mastered this, move on to matching a picture to a picture, such as finding all the pictures on flash cards that are animals, all the pictures that are food, and so on, and drop the matching pictures into the milk carton.

Use the Say What You See technique. Remember—the more you say, the more they'll learn. Notice what your child is interested in, what they are looking at, pointing at, and walking toward, and talk about what they are motivated by. Don't try to "teach" them too much or dictate what they should be interested in. Instead, keep it natural and just chat and explain what you are doing as you unload the washing machine, make lunch, or go upstairs to fetch something. Talking about everything you do will expose your child to lots of lovely new words. Remember to allow them to participate in the conversation and leave gaps for them to reply. Don't hog the conversation!

You'll notice that we're starting to implement games that require your child to sit, but what should you do when your child won't sit still to play or share storybooks, a skill that is required in preparation for school?

This is quite a common problem, but one that you do need to try to work on, as being able to sit still—along with other skills like knowing your name, holding a crayon or pencil, being able to open a book, take basic clothes off, or being potty-trained—is a desirable skill needed to start preschool.

A good way to encourage sitting and listening is to look at books, so try the following suggestions. Remember—don't put too much pressure on your child or they may refuse to play with you if they don't think it's going to be fun.

- First, ensure your child has access to several colorful board books (so that it is easy for them to turn the pages themself). Try to look at them together but allow your child to lead the flow and turn the pages, so that they are actively partaking in the activity. If they won't sit with you, flip through the book and comment on interesting pictures at a distance and let them play with it or look at it whenever they want. Initially, you could just aim to get them to sit for 2 or 3 minutes and then work toward 5 minutes.

- Help your child make their own book—a scrapbook that has things that interest them, such as photos, wrappers, artwork, stickers, and so on.

- Read bedtime stories with your child, even if they seem to be expressing more interest in carrying on playing or drinking from their sippy cup of milk. Making the effort to read them a story reinforces the idea that story time equals bedtime. Let them choose a book to read, and suggest cuddling up together. If they have a tendency to become distracted or are tired, read just one book together or say that if they come and sit down, you will read another one. Ensure the story is at the right level for your child. (See page 266 for tips on how to find the right book for your child's stage of language development.)

- During the day, pick a time when your child isn't too busy—perhaps after a nap—and just sit down on the floor and begin reading out loud. Don't worry about making them sit still on your lap. Let them run around and play while you read, if that's what they want to do. They may or may not become interested, but they are hearing you and becoming accustomed to the idea of your reading to them.

Remember—just as we adults all choose to read different books, children have different tastes, too. Why not take your child to the library and see which books interest them? If they choose a book at too high a level, go with it, but don't read the text, just talk about the pictures in a way that is one step ahead of your child's language level. So, if they are saying single words, read the book using two- or three-word sentences.

## Focusing your child's attention

Another reason that your child may not be able to sit still is if there are too many toys around. It can be difficult to focus when there is too much on offer. (This often happens to me in a cake shop—I get overexcited and want everything!) Help your child focus by putting away excess toys and, each day, bring out no more than two or three games. If they are sitting at a table to read, ensure there's nothing else within reach or in their sight line—it's always best to clear the decks.

If your child moves on to another game too soon—for example, they were doing a puzzle and moved on to the cars before finishing—quickly put most of the puzzle pieces in yourself and leave the last one or two. Then say, "First puzzle, then cars," and divert their attention back to their original choice of activity. Use phrases like "one more turn," "one more minute," and "almost finished" so that it is obvious when the game is complete.

Mealtimes can be another difficult time for sitting still. It's often tied in with eating avoidance—which, as you know, is a fairly normal part of a young child's life. My only advice here is to try not to distract your child with the TV—it's so antisocial. If things start getting frisky, give goals to work toward—for example, say, "Eat one more mouthful and then finished." If they then eat one more mouthful, don't push any more onto them unless they reach for more. Saying "Just finish your peas/carrots/potatoes" could be another thing to try.

If your child has a tendency to get down and run around at mealtimes, insist that they must sit for at least a short period. Remember that you must have high expectations! If they never sit for a meal, insist they sit for 30 seconds and then extend it. Using distractions like books or YouTube can be good for one mealtime, but it will usually become a vicious circle and the level at which you will have to distract your child will continue to increase to unsustainable levels. I used to encourage Jess to eat with a dolly, which helps symbolic play, or you could try a one-minute or two-minute egg timer and say, "You must sit for one minute and then you can get down." Give lots of praise for any attempts to sit still.

## What to do when . . . your child is saying bad words

My friend's child started speaking clearly at a very early age and was able to repeat entire sentences. The problem is that she'd learned a few embarrassing expressions (like "shut up") and she used them with strangers when they went out. My friend had tried everything to get her to stop using them—from reasoning with her to threatening to punish her—but nothing seemed to work.

If your child is using inappropriate expressions, first, ensure you are not modeling them. You may not think you are but, like me, with the "bugger" word, it wasn't until someone pointed it out that I realized how much I was saying it, so it was no wonder that Jess was saying "bu-gah," too.

Consider what might be triggering your child to say the phrase. Is it when someone unfamiliar talks to them or just when there's general noise? I met a 2-year-old child who said very little except "dit." When I asked his mum what he was saying she was embarrassed to admit that he was saying "sh*t." She explained that he'd heard her say "sh*t" when she dropped something and now said it every time he dropped something or fell over. I explained that she'd have to make a big deal of falling over at home and replacing the expletive with the word "sugar" using exactly the same tone as she would normally. Before long, her son would change "sh*t" to "sugar"!

The main advice is to try to ignore the phrase. Responding to it—and repeating it—will only make it worse. Children might be swearing to get attention. It's hard not to laugh when your child curses like a sailor, but try to remain poker-faced, as smiles and chuckles will only encourage them. Remind friends and family about this, too! They are copying what they hear from you, which, of course, we encourage at most other times in their day. Try to reset their rude words by coming up with some more interesting words altogether that won't offend but can still be used to express anger or surprise. I'm rather fond of "heck and double heck!" You may sound like a rather crazed character from an old movie, but wouldn't you rather your child was saying these harmless phrases instead of the f-word?

## Explore and encounter a range of experiences

The majority of words are learned through everyday activities, so allow your child to have a wealth of different experiences. I love this quote from professor Elizabeth Crais in the Division of Speech and Hearing Science at the University of North Carolina: "A child's knowledge of the world will be demonstrated in their word knowledge." What she's getting at is that learning to talk underpins learning and social development. The words a child uses tell us what they know about the world. Therefore, if you can expose your child to a range of experiences and talk about them in an elaborate way, this will help them to experience the world in more detail, consequently helping them to learn more. Commonly, a child might know about 4,000 to 5,000 words when they start primary school and several thousand more one year after that; the faster they learn language, the more knowledge they acquire.

Develop conversations as you go about everyday life, whether you are chatting about doing the shopping as your little one sits in the cart or telling them that Mummy is running the bath, Grandpa is cutting the grass, or Daddy is cooking. Remember to reduce your language to the right level for your child. Parents worry that they shouldn't lower their language level too much, and they try to speak in proper sentences with proper grammar. This is where being a Tuned-In Parent is crucial; you need to know at what level your child is expressing themselves by listening to them and pitching your language level slightly above. When a child reaches 4 and 5 years old you can pretty much go for it, but younger children are still learning and you need to be in tune with their level.

Expand your child's language and thought, ensuring you continue to encourage new words rather than simply repeating the words you know they can say. Have high expectations of what your child can understand and the stories they like to hear and you will see (and hear!) the rewards.

## Play Where's the . . . ?/Where's your . . . ? games

Games like this will help your child to understand that they must remember the name of the object you are saying so they can try to say it for themselves. Generally, SLPs are very critical of the approach of parents who continuously question their children because they feel it puts children off from communicating altogether (for instance, my mother-in-law continuously asked my daughter to kiss her, and Jess point-blank refused to, choosing to smother Rosa, the dog, with kisses in protest instead!). So, make the games lighthearted and fun. Give lots of praise and physically prompt your child to point at the right object if you're not sure they know. We call this error-free learning and it is a great way to keep up your child's motivation.

## Arrange playdates

The more you expose your child to other children, different toys, and new experiences, the more they will have to talk about.

## Have 10 minutes of Special Time every day

This should be uninterrupted, focused time spent being a Tuned-In Parent. During this time, observe what your child does or says and what they like to play with, and use Say What You See.

## Create a Special Time Tool Kit of resources

Fill your kit with books, pictures, toys, and treasures that your child likes. Open it each day and try to elicit language using verbal prompts. For example, you could say, "Ooh, let's see what's inside our Special Time Box today. You'd like to see the beach photos today. Look! You built a . . . with Granny and . . . and you put beautiful shells on the top. Then we ate an . . . and had a lovely swim in the . . ."

## Collect treasures

When Jess was little, I bought her a tiny chest of drawers for storing lots of tiny treasures. Jess and I filled it with a bird's feather we found in the garden, a bracelet that Gee gave her for her birthday, an injured toy Easter chick covered with dry icing so it couldn't stand up, a pine cone we found in the woods, a little rugby ball Granddad gave her when Wales won the Grand Slam, and so on. She loved listening to me telling her the stories that were associated with the objects ("Yes, this is the ball Granddad gave you. It's a lovely ball. It's a little ball with a dragon on it and the ball feels very smooth. I can throw the ball up high and catch the ball, too"). I made sure to repeat the object name over and over again—"ball," "ball." Then, when I pointed to the objects, she tried to say the words.

## Toys in the bin

Take a range of objects that belong in a particular category (e.g., animals, vehicles, etc.), say the name of the object, and drop it into a bin or a saucepan so it makes a very rewarding clunking sound. Encourage your little one to do the same.

## Books

Use a first-100-words book and take turns pointing to the things that interest your child. Joel, a little boy I am working with, loves the *Thomas the Tank Engine* first-words book—because, on every page, Thomas goes somewhere different (Joel's favorite page is the wildlife park!). I teach him the words by using his finger to point to the pictures at the side of the page, name them, then point to the same object in the busy picture. I then pause to allow him to copy me. His love of Thomas has hooked him in and encourages him to talk and exclaim with delight every time we look at the book.

Another great first-words book that features popular characters is *Richard Scarry's Best First Book Ever!*

## Repeat, repeat, repeat

Read the same stories and sing the same songs over and over again. You may get sick of the same story, but I'm certain your child won't. They will be bombarded with the vocabulary in the story and, therefore, will start to remember the words in order to use them themself. Also, if a child learns a set phrase by repetition, from a song or a book, they learn to extend their memory and learn the grammatical structures needed in sentences (we'll learn more about this in the next chapter).

## Praise every effort

Remember—praise every attempt and *don't correct*. If your child says "jamas" instead of pajamas, say, "Yes, your pajamas," and reward their efforts. Don't say, "You can only have a banana if you say it properly." Instead, try saying, "It's a . . . (banana)" and then give it whether the child says banana or not. Accept any approximation of the word and give praise. If your child says, "Ba-ba ow" when they leave the house, you say, "Bye-bye house." If you continue to correct them, you will affect their self-confidence and motivation or eagerness to want to try to communicate.

Parents often ask me if they should encourage number, shape, and color learning at an early age. My answer is that these concepts are too abstract for our little ones. Colors and numbers will come in their own time and words that carry meaning are far more useful for little ones at this age. How many times do adults use a color's name in their language? ("What a lovely pink top," or "What a beautiful red sunset.") Hardly ever—so bear that in mind. In some scenarios, knowing your colors seems to be a gauge of how clever you are, and I totally disagree with this.

## SPOTTING PROGRESS: YOU'LL KNOW YOUR EFFORTS ARE WORKING WHEN . . .

At some point, your child will no longer use an approximate word for something (for example, "duck" for bird, parrot, robin, and penguin) and will begin to spontaneously say the specific words in the correct situation, widening their vocabulary.

If your little one's use of single words isn't expanding, don't panic, don't freak out, and listen to your gut, think . . . Is my child communicating with me in other ways? Is my child motivated to communicate? Am I doing my daily Special Time to implement the strategies to help my little one?

But also make sure your gut isn't engaged in a game of one-upmanship with the mummy next door with the potty-trained 1-year-old who speaks in complete sentences on demand like a performing-monkey child. This is most definitely not "normal"!

## Chapter 6

# What to do when . . . your child isn't joining two words together

Typically, at about the age of 2 (or when a child has about 50 words), they will start to join two words together into two-word phrases. It may not surprise you to hear that some children find this quite tricky.

In order to put two words together into phrases, your child will need to be able to do the following.

- **Understand** *two* words together (such as "Mummy's cookie" or "doggy sleeping")
- **Remember** *two* words in a sequence ("give me block and dolly" when they put their toys away, for instance)
- **Express** *two* words together (such as "want toast" or "no coat"). Often the clarity of both words will diminish as the child gets their tongue around the extended syllable formation and the complexities of the new consonant sound sequence.

Think about it—that's quite an incredible leap from babbling to putting two tiny words together!

## PHRASES

A phrase is two words that we always say together. "All gone," "What's that?," "In there," "No more," "Coat on," "Shoes on," "Get down." These are considered phrases rather than two-word sentences because a child learns the whole phrase and doesn't necessarily have the ability to construct a two-word sentence for themselves yet.

Basically, a child will first learn to say single words, then some phrases appear, followed by two-word sentences that they have had to construct themself, like "Bye-bye, Kel." So, try to encourage little phrases like "Snack time!" to help your child expand the number of syllables they can put together and to guide them toward making sentences.

**Top Tip Time** **Helping the words to just pop out**

Use phrases throughout your daily routine, and to help the second word of the phrase "just pop out" of your child's mouth, leave a pause after the first word. For example, "It's time for . . . [lunch]," "Coat . . . [on]," "Open the . . . [door]," "Peeka . . . [boo]," "Ready, set . . . [go]."

## SENTENCES

Two-word sentences usually contain words from two different categories and that's why it's very important to encourage your child to become familiar with sets of words from a range of different categories (see the previous chapter). Furthermore, in order for a child's language skills to progress, a child has to fully understand what each single word means before they will attempt to put two words together. You need to be sure that your child understands your speaking to them in two-word sentences before they have a hope of saying a two-word sentence themselves. For example, do they understand "hot" and "cup" separately? If the answer's yes, then they will probably understand "hot cup" together. (To test this out, see the Top Tip Time that follows). This differs a bit from a two-word phrase, such as "all gone" or "go away" where a child might be saying two words and would not need to understand each single word component.

When your child starts attempting two-word sentences, you will also notice that they will probably attempt stories and songs using gibberish interspersed with real words. The gibberish will increase in length when your child cannot think of the right word. For instance, I spotted my little girl saying a stream of gibberish and then putting her fingers in her mouth to say "pop" and I knew instantly that she was trying to sing "Pop Goes the Weasel."

## How two-word sentences usually start to appear

There is a loose developmental pattern relating to the order in which two-word sentences appear. This is listed here.

1. "That" *plus* object: "that car," "that duck"

2. "More" *plus* action or object: "more hide," "more splashing," "more book," "more cake"

3. "No" and disappearance/nonexistence *plus* object, person, or action: "no sleep," "Mummy gone," "no raisins"

4. Person *plus* object: "Daddy cake," "Harry shoe"

5. Concept *plus* object/person: "little flower," "dirty feet," "cold yogurt," "hot potato"

6. Possessive pronoun/"belonging" word *plus* object or person: "my granddad," "Mummy plate"

7. Object or person *plus* action: "baby cry," "Daddy dig," "bird up," "cat meow"

8. Action/object/person *plus* location word: "climb in," "go down," "fall out," "on nose," "cat in"

9. Question word *plus* object or person: "where Mummy?," "who that?"

To encourage your child's first two-word sentence, let's first go back to boosting their understanding.

**Top Tip Time** **Understanding two-word sentences**

Once our children start to talk, we are desperate for them to say more and more, seeking to get inside their minds and draw out their thoughts and feelings about the world. The first step toward this is to encourage your child to understand two-word sentences. Once they have achieved this, they'll attempt to use them. Try the following techniques.

- Gather the following objects—apple, banana, cookie, teddy, and dolly (or use two favorite cuddly toys). Sit the teddy and dolly down in front of your child with the apple, banana, and cookie. Ask them to "Give teddy the cookie" and "Give dolly the apple." If they do not understand, repeat the instruction and demonstrate the activity for them.

- Find a sponge, a teddy, and a doll. Give the sponge to your child and ask them to "Wash teddy's leg" or "Wash dolly's hair." As previously stated, if your child does not understand, repeat the instruction and demonstrate the activity for them.

- Find a box and a basket, or a barn and a house, and gather some objects, animals, or people. Ask your child to "put the cow in the barn," "put the dog in the basket" and "put the spoon in the house." Now swap roles and see if your child will direct you to hide the objects.

- Make a mailbox out of an old shoebox. Make some flash cards of people doing things from pictures from a catalog— for example, man sleeping, girl running, and so on. Say the sentence out loud and see if your child knows which picture you are talking about. Encourage them to describe the picture by starting them off with "It's a . . ."

- We have talked a lot about giving choices, so now begin to give choices at a two-word level. When your child is reaching for more raisins and you know exactly what they want, plead ignorance and say, "More orange or more raisins?" Don't always anticipate your child's needs—make them work a bit harder to communicate what they want or need by talking.

- Try to ensure that older siblings aren't doing all the talking. Give your younger child an opportunity to speak, even if they say nothing. (Read more advice on dealing with older siblings, page 260.)

- Use the Copy and Add technique. Every time your child says a sound or a word you should copy the word and add another word. So, Ewan says, "Grapes" and you say, "Yummy grapes"; Hope says, "Car" and you say, "Fast car"; Noah says, "Mummy" and you say, "Mummy's eating," and so on. Try doing this whenever your child utters a sound, a word, and later, when they say a sentence.

- Play enjoyable games with your child—bubbles are always fun and I make sure I always have a bottle of bubble mixture at my clinic, and in my handbag for that matter! Blow some bubbles for your child and let them pop. If they say, "Pop," say, "Bubbles pop," or if they say, "Bubble," you say, "More bubbles" or "I want bubbles." Make "big bubbles," "small bubbles," blow "bubbles up" or "bubbles down" in order to expand their understanding of two-word sentences. It's simple to do and yet it can have such a positive effect. Other fun games will also elicit a request for more—"more slide," "splash again," "more balloons" and "tickle again," for instance.

- At this phase, if Jess ever saw someone go or heard someone say, "Bye," we played a turn-taking game where she said, "Bye," and I added a name onto the end. It goes like this.

    Jess: "Ba."

    Me: "Bye, Lyn."

    Jess: "Ba."

    Me: "Bye, William."

    Jess: "Ba."

Me: "Bye, Uncle Stevo."

As you can imagine, this game goes on for quite some time—it's nearly as popular with Jess as peekaboo!

- Practice greeting people and things—take things out of the toy box and say, "Hello, teddy," "Hello, book," "Hello, train," and so on. And when you see people, encourage your child to say hello, too. This is good on the phone.

- If you have one of those pop-up games in which animals or people pop up when you push a button, say, "Farmer up," "Cow up," "Sheep up," and then say, "Sheep down," "Cow down" as you push them down.

- Place objects into a shape sorter and say, "Bye, block," "Block gone," etc.

- Play hiding games—get a dish towel and hide things under it, then say, "Teddy's gone" or "Car's gone."

- Make a "gone" book—a book that has an object on one page and nothing (a blank page) on the next. So, you can say "ball," then "ball's gone," and so on. Encourage your child to say, "Bed's gone," and not just "gone," as you would've expected in the previous phase.

- Involve your child in simple chores like loading the washing machine, and explain what you are doing—"Socks in," "Tights in," and so on.

- Point to parts of the body and say, "Cari's nose," "Cari's tummy." Labeling body parts is a good way to start introducing two-word sentences.

- Your child should be able to hum and sing, so encourage them to sing two words at the end of a sentence rather than just one—for example, at the end of "Twinkle, twinkle," your child might sing, "little star." (See tips on how to encourage words through song, page 67.)

- Your child will also be learning how to express pain verbally, so model sentences like "Hurt my finger" or "Sore bottom." You can role-play this with cuddly toys falling over or going to the doctor. Consider purchasing a doctor's kit, which is a great learning prop.

- Watch TV together and talk about and act out the programs using two-word sentences, such as "Elmo's crying," "Big Bird's cuddling," and "Peppa's lost; where's Peppa? In the box."
- Use role-play scenarios involving appropriate two-word comments. So, if you were playing shopping you might say, "Buy the bread." If you were pretending to be at the dentist, say, "Mouth open," or, if you're pretending to give dolly a bath, say, "Wash her neck."

## AND, ACTION! HELLO, VERBS

The first set of words your little one will learn to say tend to be names of people (Mummy, sister), names of objects (favorite toys or food), social words (hello, bye-bye, night-night), and describing words (hot, cold, dirty, big). It's exciting! And, once they have a selection of each (about 50 words in total), they start to add the noun to the verb to build a small sentence—"Mummy sleeping," "Teddy walking," "Brushing teeth," and so on.

Some children need to be encouraged to use verbs once they have a stream of nouns and may use very general words that they apply to everything, such as "get" and "do" in place of more specific verbs. So, your child might say "doing bricks" rather than "building bricks" or "get up" rather than "climb up the ladder."

**Top Tip Time** **Helping your child to learn new verbs**

Children need to understand the meaning of a verb before they'll say it, so these games use repetition, simplified language and real-life experiences to cement their understanding and encourage them to vocalize their growing list of action words. And you won't even have to make a conscious effort to "learn" most of them because they just revolve around daily life.

## Say What You See

Think about your child's daily life and what they actually do. A typical morning probably goes something like this: Get up, snuggle in bed, change nappy, carry downstairs, drink milk, get dressed, watch TV, eat breakfast, and so on. This is where my Say What You See technique is invaluable—repeat as many of the action words as possible—"Changing your nappy," "Drinking milk," "Getting dressed," etc.

When watching TV or reading books, point out to your child what people/animals are doing: "Look—Zac's jumping," "Mummy's cooking," "Dolly is dancing," "Spot's eating," and so on.

You can use the same technique while playing with your child: "Teddy falling," "Dolly crying," "Dog drinking."

## Scrapbook

Make a scrapbook of family members doing things, or collect magazine pictures of people doing things—painting, laughing, kicking, eating—and say each action as you look at the pictures.

## Naming games

Collect pictures from magazines of people or animals performing activities, then create a game where your child tells you what they are all doing. You could even make a mailbox out of an old shoebox (simply cut a rectangular mail slot in it) so your child can put the pictures into it. I often use this game at my clinic because children love trying to cut and push the mail through the mailbox slot, and it makes learning verbs fun for them.

Hide the pictures around the room and ask your child to find a particular one: "Where's . . . sleeping?"—do the sign to help. (It is always useful to go back to signs when you are teaching your child new words, particularly verbs and prepositions [positional words]. Signs provide visual information to back up the spoken word, making it easier to retain.)

## Act up

Act out as many of the actions as possible and encourage your child to copy you to help them understand the meaning of the verb.

Embarrassingly, when my daughter was getting fussy—particularly when waiting for her breakfast—I often found myself leaping around the kitchen performing actions for her and saying, "Mummy's dancing," "Mummy's kicking," "Mummy's singing," "Mummy's spinning!" while trying to butter her toast at the same time. Slightly bonkers, but very effective for language development and for avoiding meltdowns!

## Other games that encourage word combining

- Take two sets of objects or pictures, mix them up, and then sort them. For example, try food versus animals—put the food into a toy shopping cart and the animals into a barn.
- Make a scrapbook of pictures of objects cut out from a magazine, with a different set of objects on each page.
- Make a slideshow of photos for your iPad that feature a particular topic, such as garden words, nursery words, or food words.

---

### 5 ADDITIONAL WAYS TO PROMOTE COMMUNICATION . . . IN A RESTAURANT

1. **Disappearing Act:** Have your child examine the objects on the table. Ask them to hide their eyes, and take one object away. Ask them to remember what has gone. Repeat with multiple objects.

2. **Telephone:** Send a whispered message around the table and see if it's the same at the end.

3. **Salty Sounds:** Pour a little salt on the table and write a letter in it. Then look for an object in the room that starts with that sound.

---

4. **Blind Taste Test:** Put a piece of food in your child's mouth and ask them to guess what it is by tasting and not looking. Encourage lots of lovely describing words like "sweet," "sticky," etc.

5. **Charades:** One of our favorite family games is to deliver the dessert menu by acting. Try it out—it's easier than you think.

## Writing a word list

It's obviously hard to keep track of how many words your child knows so it might be an idea to start keeping a list—don't just write down the word but write down the way your child says it. This will help you to keep one step ahead of them and it's also really rewarding for you to see your child's progress! (And it's fun to look back and reminisce about them later on, too.)

## Please and thank you dilemmas!

Don't worry too much about teaching your child to say "please" and "thank you." When you know only 50 words, it's far better that they be functional words that carry a message. Only once your child can put a short sentence together should you then add the social niceties.

When my daughter, Jess, was little she started saying "Ah" and pointing at everything she wanted. When I picked her up from my mother's house one day, my mother said, "I'll encourage her to say 'please' instead." I had to tell her that this is a real no-no. We didn't want Jess to say "please" thinking that *please* is a better word for drink, book, outside, etc., because she'd then end up saying, "Please please!"

I discussed this issue with one of my speech therapy friends, Katie, who had taught her son George lots of single words and signs and was not worried about "please" and "thank you." She said it was quite embarrassing when George would go up to an adult and say, "Drink!" because he was too young to say the two-word sentence "Drink, please." This left Katie worrying about whether or not other people thought she was a terrible mother for not encouraging George to say please and thank you. I'd still argue that there's plenty of time to learn these social graces and that for now, it's far better to have functional words that will help your child communicate their needs.

Going to baby groups and meeting mummy friends is one of the hardest times, when you're secretly thinking, "My little peach doesn't have as many words as they do." You may find yourself wondering if everything's okay and really hoping that things will pick up soon. Perhaps you have a child who seems to communicate well but doesn't vocalize as you would expect. Perhaps you're wondering whether there's anything more suspicious going on, knowing that they had a lot of coughs, colds, and sniffles since starting nursery school a few months ago.

If you have these concerns, ask a professional for some reassurance and have a Special Time plan in place using the Top Tip times to help. You'll start to feel so much better if you take positive action—I'm sure of it.

# Chapter 7

# What to do when . . . your child's speech is difficult to understand

When your child starts to blend words together, they will probably use a repeated single syllable (for example, "baba" for "baby," "nana" for "banana," "gangan" for "granny"), and much of what they say will be difficult to understand because their consonant sounds aren't quite right. The first consonant might be incorrect ("dat" for "cat" or "dacda" for "tractor") and the last not there at all ("uh" for "up" or "buh" for "bus"), but the vowels should be almost perfect by now, which will help you to work out what the target word is. And when your child begins to blend two words together, the clarity of both the words will decrease even though previously the clarity of both single words was okay! This is because the complexity of the whole utterance has increased.

Some of your child's attempts at words will make you laugh out loud. (I've often heard "Winnie the Pooh" spoken as "ne dah poo" by little ones, or heard "cwock" for "clock"!) And because of the way your little one says a word in such a unique and cute way, your whole family might take on that word and use it for years to come. For example, we may sound crazy to strangers but, in our house, we all say, "Tupatupatea" for "Cup of tea," "Coo me" for "Excuse me," and "nin-nins" for "raisins."

My father was so eager to have a unique word for "Granddad" that he didn't refer to himself as anything and waited to see what his grandson would come up with. He's now known as "Geedad."

Your child's speech may be slightly unclear but you'll understand most of it because, hopefully, you're so tuned in to their favorite toys and games and the experiences they have that you'll know what they're going to say even before they say it. Strangers, though, won't be quite so up to speed with their lingo, so you'll probably end up doing a fair bit of interpreting—for instance, strangers are thought to understand the chatter of a 2-year-old only about 50 percent of the time.

For this reason, let's start thinking about how you can encourage your little one to improve the clarity of their speech by teaching them to listen to the sounds that make up words. You have to listen to and decode sequences of sounds in words before you can have a chance of saying those words. This is known as phonological awareness and phonological processing.

## GETTING SOME CLARITY

It takes time to master the ability to string a bunch of speech sounds together to make a word. As we've learned, vowel sounds are the easiest sounds to make, and then there's a pattern to how consonant sounds develop.

We take our speech and language skills for granted (speech being the sounds that make up words, and language being the words that make up sentences), but can you imagine how difficult it is for a toddler to talk? Every single new word that passes their lips is like one tremendously challenging tongue-twister. So, you won't be shocked when I tell you that clear speech will take time and a lot of practice—and some people never manage it!

Your child probably leaves off the ends of words and the beginnings of words and uses alternative consonant sounds. If their errors are consistent, you may not notice this so much because you'll be tuned in to the way they talk, but if you try writing down a few of their words, you'll start noticing the patterns of their errors, and some may even make you giggle.

Don't worry—this is your child's very clever built-in editing system. It's essentially their way of simplifying words down to their most basic form so they can try to say them. In time, with lots of word modeling from you, and practice and repetition from them, they will hopefully start to say words more clearly and unfamiliar adults won't look to you to interpret for them.

It is important to applaud your child for their efforts and revel in their wonderful attempts at tongue-twisting challenges, like "animal," "helicopter," and "hospital," which will probably sound more like "aminal," "topter," and "hopital"!

## Your child will probably simplify language in the following ways

- **Reduplication:** This is repetition of the same syllable to make a word; for example, "daddy" becomes "dada," "water" is said as "wawa," "Elmo" becomes "momo."
- **Weak syllable deletion:** In a word there is often a weak syllable (for instance, "gu" in "guitar") and a child will delete it. "Guitar" becomes "tar," "spaghetti" becomes "getti."
- **Final consonant deletion:** for example, "buh" for "bus," "uh" for "up."
- **Cluster reduction:** Many words have two consonant sounds that are positioned next to one another. This is called a consonant cluster. Blending two sounds into a consonant cluster is very difficult for a young child to do, and therefore, they might drop one of the sounds completely—for example, "FLower" = "fower," "GRanny" = "gangan," "SPoon" = "poon," "STar" = "tar."
- **Fronting:** Some sounds are articulated with your lips ("p," "b," "m") and others with your tongue. Some use the tongue tip ("t," "d," "n") and others use the back of the tongue

("k," "g"). The sounds articulated with the back of your tongue are harder to say, and it is very common for children to misarticulate these sounds. Instead, they tend to replace them with the tongue-tip sounds. So, "cow" will be "tow," "car" will be "tar," and "gate" will be "date."

- **Gliding:** This refers to replacement of the consonants "l" and "r" with the consonants "y" and "w" so that "lion" is pronounced as "yion" and "rabbit" as "wabbit."

- **Assimilation, or consonant harmony:** The child uses the same consonant twice to make the word easier to say, so, for example, "dog" becomes "gog," and "yellow" becomes "lellow."

It's a wonder any child ever gets the word right when they have all these "processes" to contend with! But rest assured—over time, your child's speech will get clearer and clearer the more a word is modeled and the more they attempt to say it.

## CASE STUDY: WAYBAJEA!— TRACEY AND MINNIE

When Tracey's daughter Minnie was around 2 years old, she began shouting, "Waybajea!" whenever she was excited or something good had happened. Tracey was a bit confused but thought it might be something that was said at nursery school or a lyric from a song that she didn't know. This went on for quite a few weeks before Tracey was watching a TV show called *Something Special* with Minnie and noticed that the presenter Justin Fletcher (aka Mr. Tumble) was encouraging the children to "wave or cheer" when they spotted a cat. Minnie shouted, "Waybajea!" when she saw the cat, and the penny dropped. She was saying her interpretation of "wave or cheer." Tracey said, "Yes, the cat, let's wave or cheer!," speaking very clearly to model the words correctly, and after a few repetitions Minnie had it nailed.

# LISTENING FOR SPEECH SOUNDS

We are hearing and listening continuously, but is the brain actively engaged in what it is listening to? Possibly not, and, consequently, some children need help to learn to listen to the sounds that make up a word before they can learn to say the sound in order to speak clearly.

Hearing is a passive process that involves the ear simply hearing sounds. On the other hand, listening is an active process that involves tuning in, decoding, and responding to sounds in the environment. It sounds rather silly, but you need to train your ear to hear in order to listen—which is pretty difficult in a world that often involves continuous background noise like the TV and radio, or constant chatter at nursery school. The ability to listen to speech sounds is fundamental to speech and language development. In the speech therapy world, this is known as phonological awareness.

Your brain must not only listen to and process the single sounds that make up a word but also decode a whole word to determine if it recognizes the pattern of sounds together and the sequence in which that word appears (its context within a grammatical sentence). It is said that we retain the whole sentence in our working memory before we process it. This whole system is known as auditory processing.

As we've already learned, you can expect a range of different mistakes in your child's speech, but they go through the same developmental pattern of learning sounds—the first consonant sounds you'll hear are "p," "b," "m, "d," "h," and "n" in place at the beginning of a word ("pig," "bee," "milk," "dog," "house," and "no"), then "k," "g," "t," "n," "ng" next. The use of all consonants at the end or in the middle of words will be erratic. Therefore, your child will have to listen to these sounds when you model them within words. If they are not using one of these sounds, they may need to be encouraged to listen to the sound in order to help them say it.

**Top Tip Time** **Honing those listening skills**

The games listed below are designed to be fun and entertaining and to help your child focus their attention on the sounds that make up words. By encouraging your child to have excellent phonological awareness (see page 138) you will be preparing them for reading and writing, so whatever level your child is at—whether they're saying 20 or 200 words), there's no harm in giving these exercises a try. Some of the games may seem familiar, which is because they are games I've suggested previously, but they are taken to the next level. Always remember that if your child says the sound incorrectly, reward their attempt, then simply model the correct target for them (see a full explanation on how to model words for your child on page 82).

### Create a sound sack

Make up a bag of objects that start with one particular sound and encourage your child to pull them out and name each one. Why not make a sound sack for a range of different sounds? Initially focus on the sounds that you know your child should be able to say by the end of this phase—"p," "b," "m," "h," "n," and "d." So, in a "b" sack you would put a ball, bed, boy, bear, bus, block, or book, and in an "m" sack you would put a monkey, money, man, moon, or mouse. Move on to the sounds your child is struggling with. Encourage your child to listen to the target sound by emphasizing it clearly to them.

### Read, read, read!

One of the best ways to help children naturally develop an awareness of speech sounds (otherwise known as phoneme awareness) is through the use of children's books, so look out for stories that rhyme, use alliteration, or have some sort of predictable pattern— for example, *Each Peach Pear Plum*. This type of awareness is a very important milestone in the development of early literacy.

Being aware of rhyme is important when learning to read and spell because it can help children appreciate that words that share common sounds often share common letter sequences. So, if you can spell "hat," you can also spell "bat," "rat," and "mat." This also applies to reading: if you can read "call," you can read "ball," "tall," and "fall."

Being able to recognize rhyming words helps the child develop the ability to break down longer words into smaller parts and then recognize those smaller parts (for example, "call," then "calling" and "called"). Again, this is an important skill for reading and spelling. Reread stories over and over again, allowing children to occasionally "fill in the blanks" with an appropriate rhyming word.

### Get rhyming

Make up some rhymes of your own and try to act them out. You could make an airplane fly in the sky, for example. Leave pauses so that your child can add in the missing word. Below are some ideas to get you started.

- Fly in the . . . (sky)
- Sheep is . . . (asleep)
- Mouse in a . . . (house)
- Duck on a . . . (truck)
- A bee in the . . . (tree)
- Sing on a . . . (swing)

Remember that singing songs makes language stick, so perhaps sing these sentences in a song. Try singing to the tune to "If You're Happy and You Know It" for "There's a fly in the sky, way up high," for instance.

Make up rhyming nicknames for friends and family, such as Stevie Weavie, Sally Mally, Cam Wham, or Pat Cat. Why? Because children love to do this! One child I worked with said, "Listen to my song," and came out with a list of rhyming words.

## Hit the mic!

Use an echo mic from a toy shop or a real microphone to practice saying some individual speech sounds or rhyming words. You could say, "What is the next word?" then hold the mic next to your child's mouth. For example, with "Humpty Dumpty," sing: "Humpty Dumpty sat on a wall, Humpty Dumpty had a great . . . [hold up the mic to your little one]."

Or try singing nursery rhymes and alter them so that your child can learn to tell the difference and discriminate the first sounds of the word, then correct you. For example, try "Little Bo Peep has lost her jeep," "Jack and Jill went up the mill," and "Hickory dickory dock, the mouse ran up the rock."

## Play puppets

Make a puppet say a sound and ask your child to copy it—for example, try "furry Fred says 'fff.' Can you say it, too?" Make the puppet ask for things but get it wrong so your child has to correct him—for instance, "I want my chook" (book) and "Give me a dink" (drink). Your child can use the context to determine what furry Fred means. Then have the puppet repeat the rhyming words (and maybe even add one more)—for example, a puppet that can only say words that sound like "drink": "think," "wink," "sink," "mink," "link."

## Domestic noises

Listen to household noises and make them into speech sounds. Your child may be able to name the object, but they may need to be encouraged to broaden their use of speech sounds. For instance, they may say "bish" for "fish," so if you encourage them to say the "f" sound away from the word "fish," they should begin to transfer the skills they have learned in order to say "f" correctly on its own and in real words. For other sounds, try vacuum cleaner = v v v; rain = t t t; boiling teakettle = f f f; wind = w w w; dishwasher = sh sh sh; bouncing ball = b b b.

## Identifying which speech sounds your child is struggling with

The best way to do this is to use a picture book and ask your child to label simple pictures. Write down how they say the words and see if a pattern emerges.

Once you've established which speech sounds your child is struggling to say, try the following tricks to help them say that sound. I've listed the sounds that most commonly cause problems and suggested games that may help (see pages 143–44). It's a good idea to practice these exercises in the mirror so that your child can see what their mouth is doing. Remember to encourage them, even if they don't say the correct sound. Don't let it become a negative experience for them—it's supposed to be fun!

## SMOOTHING OUT THE TRICKIER SPEECH SOUNDS

It's when your child begins to "freestyle," chatting away about anything and everything (whether it's in the here and now or a creation from their imagination), that you may start to notice some quirks in their speech. After all, they are still fairly new to speech, so it's only natural that they are still refining their sounds and words.

For example, when Minnie was little, Tracey noticed that she had a bit of an issue with saying the "l" sound after another consonant, and was using "w" instead. So, "clock" was "cwock," "play" was "pway," and "flag" was "fwag," despite her being able to pronounce the "l" sound (she could say "lion" and "lemonade").

This is perfectly normal for a young child. Try not to become too panicked by a speech-sound error, as all sounds have a developmental pattern and the error your child is making may be completely in sync for the level of their spoken language. Look at the guidelines below to help you decipher whether your child should have a particular sound or not at a particular stage of their

142

development. With Minnie, we knew that she *could* say "l" so, in time, she would manage to blend two consonant sounds together (such as "cl," "pl," or "fl") so that her speech would sound perfect!

Although Tracey initially feared this might be a long-standing habit, I was able to reassure her that this is totally fine—and temporary. After a month or two of playing the Top Tip Time games aimed at perfecting speech sounds for about 5 minutes on most days, Minnie started to get her consonant blends right, although Tracey still noticed that the error crept in when Minnie was tired.

On a different note, my brother has Down syndrome. One of his friends who also has it talks a lot but is difficult to understand. I know that Stevo's friend would benefit hugely from some speech-sound work, and I know that even though he's in his 30s, it would work!

## Common speech-sound errors

In order to offer the same reassurance to as many parents as I can, the following is my list of common speech-sound "bumps" that become apparent at around this time. See which ones you recognize from your little one's chatter.

- Your child may be mixing up their *d*'s, *g*'s, *t*'s and *c/k*'s, so you might hear "dog" as "gog" and "car" as "tar." This should improve at about 3 years of age.
- "Sh," "ch," "j," and "jz" will be difficult at this age (sh = shoe, ch = chocolate, j = jam and jz found in television). You will hear "shop" as "sop," "chip" as "tyip," and "jelly" as "delly."
- "R" will be articulated as "w," so "rabbit" becomes "wabbit."
- "L" is likely to be articulated as "y," so "lion" becomes "yion."
- Your child will definitely not be able to say "z," "th," and "v," so "zoo" becomes "soo" or "doo," "three" becomes "free," and "van" is "ban" or "fan."

- At 2 years, a child will regularly leave the final sound off a word (so "buh" for "bus" or "uh" for "up," for instance), while at 2½ years, a middle or final consonant might be inserted, but it will often be incorrect (so, "but" for "bus" or "ub" for "up"). If the target sound has been achieved at the start of the word, then it is only a matter of time until that sound appears in the middle and the end of the word.
- You will also hear many muddled words, such as "hopital" for "hospital," "aminal" for "animal," "elemy" for "Emily," or "diccifult" for "difficult"—all normal!
- If you have any concerns about any of the above, below are some Top Tip Time games that aim to tackle each common issue.

**Top Tip Time** **Let's sort the speech sounds**

Young children learn words as a whole and are not generally aware that a word is made up of a sequence of separate sounds. It's only if a child has pronunciation difficulties that we have to break down the word into each component to make it easier for them to become aware of the sounds. This has to be done first through discriminating between the target sound and the articulated sound, and then rebuilding the target sound into the word by articulating the single sound, then saying a sound with a vowel, then that sound in a word.

I hope this doesn't all sound too much like homework. I want this section to reassure you about what's normal and empower you to confidently help your child without lessening their enthusiasm for talking. By focusing on one target consonant speech sound at a time, their speech sounds will improve. Let's take a child who is continuously replacing "f" for "b"—for instance, saying "bish" instead of "fish." In order to correct this you have to teach them to say "ffff" on its own (biting your bottom lip with your top teeth like a rabbit), then "fff" plus a vowel (e.g., "fee, fi, fo, fum"), then real words beginning with "fff," such as "fan," "fair," "farm," "forest," and so on, and finally "fff" words in sentences. Let them take their time and learn slowly, and keep practicing the target sound, even after they have learned to say it, so they can fine-tune their new speech sound into a word.

## The kit

Invest in a set of picture sound cards that represent a whole range of sounds. (There are many varieties—Jolly Phonics Cards are probably the most well known.) These are sets of cards, each with a picture and possibly a letter on it. The picture is usually something that represents the sound (for instance, a snake for an "s" sound or a baby sleeping for the "sh" sound). Use these cards to encourage your child to say the sounds they find tricky. Remember—if the letter is written on the card, always use the sound and not the letter name (so for the letter *s* you would say "ssssss," not "ess").

## Stage 1: Listening to the difference in sounds

Your child needs to be able to distinguish between the target sound and the incorrect sound. For example, if they say "dun" for "sun," you'll use pictures that represent "s" and "d" to check that they can hear the difference between the two sounds. You will say those sounds randomly and encourage them to point to the corresponding sound card (they should manage this from a selection of four or five sound cards at about 2½ years). You could vary this activity by encouraging your child to stick a sticker on the correct sound card or throw a beanbag onto it.

You have now established whether or not your child can discriminate between the incorrect and target sounds. They cannot move on to the next stage until they are able. Once you know your child can make the distinction, help them to cement this understanding. For instance, in the *s* example above, in which the child replaces an "s" sound with a "d" sound, you could emphasize the fact that the "s" sound is a long sound and the "d" sound is a short sound.

If your child is unable to discriminate between the sounds, have their hearing assessed—if they can't hear sounds, they certainly won't say them. If their hearing has been checked, play the listening games on pages 60–63 to help them improve their listening skills.

Totally immerse your child in the sounds they are finding tricky. This is known as auditory bombardment and involves saying the target sound almost continuously during everyday experiences to help the child hear it. So, using our "sun" example, you'd find as many opportunities as possible to say "sss." So if you're threading beads, say "sss" as the beads are whizzing down the string; say "sss" when you are sizzling sausages on the stove; say "sss" when an evil character comes on TV; and say "sss" when wiping the table as you make a snake shape with the cloth.

Some sounds are particularly hard, such as "k" or "c." When this is the case, it is very important not to put pressure on your child to say the sound. Instead, play a range of listening games to let them hear the sound while you say it—over and over again, until you're blue in the face!

## Stage 2: Producing the single sound

In this stage you help your child to practice saying the target sound on its own—using our example, it would be the "s" sound. This will be very easy for some children, but others will need lots of adult help before they can do it (see tips on finessing speech sounds).

You could try to

- draw the sound and the picture that represents it,
- make a Play-Doh model of an object associated with the sound "s"—for example, a snake or a snail,
- say "s" as you place the "s" sound card into a homemade mailbox,
- place a number of "s" sound cards against bowling pins and knock them down,

- use the "s" sound cards as stepping stones and say them out loud, and/or
- play I Spy . . . choosing anything beginning with "s."

## Stage 3: Blending the target sound with a vowel to make a "silly" word

This is the pre-real-word stage. So, you might try blending "s-oo"/"s-ee"/"s-ah." This is all done using picture sound cards to represent the consonant and the vowel sounds (e.g., a snake for "sss" and a mouse for "ee," or a ghost for "ooo." I usually place the consonant sound card next to the vowel card and blend them—"s" and "ooo" (snake plus ghost sound cards) make "sooo." The aim is to get the two sounds blending smoothly, but to begin with, there might be a gap between the target sound and the vowel—this is okay.

You could also try stacking vowel cards next to bowling pins and asking your little one to throw the ball at them. Whichever pin they knock down, take the vowel picture and match it to the tricky consonant—I place the consonant next to the right side of my mouth and the vowel next to the left and move my head from right to left as I say the sounds "sss" and "ooo" so that the child is directed to look at the pictures and can see how my mouth moves at the same time.

At this age, children enjoy playing with language and words (for example, whispering and copying varying intonation patterns), so you could find a puppet and make it say all of these rather random words as you blend the target consonant sound with a vowel.

## Stage 4: Saying really short words!

When a child is able to blend the consonant and the vowel sound together really smoothly (as in Stage 3), they are ready to try short words. Use pictures of objects that begin with the target sound (following our "s" example, this could be sea, sock, sun, sand, Sam, and sad). Play the games that follow to practice saying these short words. Avoid words that have a two-consonant blend at the beginning, such as spider, slide, swim and star, as these are much harder to say than words in which there is a consonant followed by a vowel. Always remember to reward your child's efforts and model the word correctly if they say it wrong.

Go around the house and collect objects that begin with your sound. Put them into a sound sack as you encourage your child to say the words.

- Make two identical sets of picture cards using two identical catalogs. Pick out the cards showing objects beginning with your target letter. You could play a pairing game. In Snap, often the first card game that children learn, you deal out a pack of picture cards and take turns putting them facedown. When someone puts down a card that matches the previous one, the first person to shout, "Snap!" gets to take the whole pile of cards. The person who ends up with all the cards is the winner.

- Play the Tray Game, in which you have a number of objects or pictures of objects starting with the target sound on a tray, then you cover them and take one away. Your child has to remember which object or picture has been removed and try to say the word.

- Make a slideshow of pictures starting with a particular sound using Google Images and go through them with your child using your laptop or iPad.

- Write a list of foods starting with the target sound and go shopping for them together. Working with the "s" example, you could look for sausages, steak, salami, cereal (think first *sound*, not first letter), celery, cilantro, sandwich, salad, and squash.

- Hide "s" pictures around the room and ask your child to find them and encourage all of your child's efforts to say the words as they identify the pictures they have found.

- Finishing a word or phrase in a storybook works really well, too. Go to the library or just raid your own books to find stories with characters whose names start with the target letter. So, for our "s" example, *Where's Spot?* would work well.

• Make a scrapbook of pictures that begin with the target sound—"My 's' book"—using pictures from magazines and catalogs. Or choose a range of sounds and have a page for "s," a page for "d," and so on.

If your child is struggling with a word, say it with them and emphasize the target sound—"ssssock." Don't get them to try too many times if it's really difficult for them—it creates a real sense of negativity. In such a case, it's useful to go back to Stage 3.

## Stage 5: Short phrases

When your child is able to say short words, we move on to putting the words into a short phrase. (It's better when the word starting with the target letter is the second word in the sentence as this is representative of how the target word would appear in a longer sentence—i.e., next to another sound.) So, with the "s" example, you could try phrases such as "big sun," "blue sock," and "red saw."

You could draw a number of socks on a page, color each one a different color, then practice saying, "Blue sock," "Red sock," and so on. This is more difficult than it sounds and your child will often need help to know when they need to say the target sound at the beginning of the second word. Sometimes, a child will say the target letter at the beginning of both words (so, using the "s" example, "sssblue sssock"). If this happens, encourage them to listen carefully to establish which of the words starts with the snake noise, and ask, "Does 'blue' start with 's'? No, it starts with 'b.' Let's try again. B-lue sssock." (I often use the snake sign to visually prompt the child into saying "s" in the correct place.)

## Stage 6: Putting the target word in a sentence

When a child is able to use short phrases with target words, encourage them to then think of a sentence to use the word in—for example, "The sun is in the sky."

- This can be done using storybooks, particularly if they revolve around a character whose name begins with the target letter (working with the "s" example, Spot in *Where's Spot?* and other books by Eric Hill) or around a subject that starts with the target letter (for "s," it could be a story about swimming, sun, sea, and sand or school).

- When you go out, look for things that begin with the target letter and talk about them (for instance, "Let's tell Daddy what that naughty seagull did").

- Use the target letter in general conversation, too—this can be difficult, because it's hard for children when they are trying so hard to tell you something and are in a rush to remember to use that blasted "s" word. Remember that the words that have been spoken incorrectly for the longest time (the earliest and possibly most frequently occurring words) will be the last to change—old habits die hard. My advice is to tell your child, "From now until we get to the store (no more than 5 minutes) we're going to try really hard to say the "s" sound."

- You should also ensure that a high-frequency word, such as "sock," is always spoken clearly. Focus on another three or four words starting with that sound. If one word is consistently spoken correctly, others will also slip into place. Your child should be able to say this word correctly within a sentence before you move on to the next stage.

- Get your child to try tongue-twisters to develop speech sounds at a sentence length. My favorites include the following.

  » *Cooks cook cupcakes quickly*

  » *Flora's freshly fried flying fish*

  » *Purple paper people*

  » *She sells seashells by the seashore*

  » *I scream, you scream, we all scream for ice cream!*

  » *Peter Piper picked a peck of pickled peppers,*
     *If Peter Piper picked a peck of pickled peppers,*
     *Where's the peck of pickled peppers Peter Piper picked?*

» *I thought a thought.*

*But the thought I thought wasn't the thought I thought I thought.*

*If the thought I thought I thought had been the thought I thought, I wouldn't have thought so.*

» *I saw a saw that could out-saw any other saw I ever saw.*

## Stage 7: Using the sound in other places or in different positions within words

When your toddler has mastered the previous stages and can say the target sound at the beginning of the word, it's more than likely that, given a bit of time, the sound will be spoken correctly across all positions in a word. If this doesn't happen, you need to go back to Stage 3 and work up to Stage 7 again, putting the target sound at the end of a word, or within a phrase, as in Stage 5.

## Stage 8: Blending two consonants together

Blends are difficult to articulate and may need a lot of practice. Generally, we do not worry about whether a child can say blends until they reach at least 4½ or 5 years of age.

You will need some new pictures of words that begin with your target consonant sound blended with another consonant. So, working with the "s" example, these will be "sl," "st," "sm," "sn," "sw," and "sk." Make each blend the new target sound and start back at Stage 2, getting your child to say the blend on its own, and progress from there.

## Points to remember

If your child is not saying the sound correctly after two or possibly three tries (you know your child's limits better than I do), keep praising them and back off (this is the case from Stage 2 onward). After this number of attempts, they are probably not ready to say the sound or word correctly.

- In general conversation, again, allow your child two or three attempts and then give up as, after this many attempts, you are unlikely to understand the word they are attempting to say. Try to take the pressure off by encouraging them to show you or somehow give you a clue. If it becomes too frustrating for them, distract them by changing the subject completely (for instance, "Did I tell you I saw Bob the Builder today?").

- Don't correct a child all the time—it's too intense and your child will get annoyed and may not want to play with you anymore. Choose a five-minute slot in your day to practice or choose one single word that you are going to focus on.

- Always keep in mind that your child is doing their best, not being lazy (I hear this complaint *a lot*). I know that children always communicate to the best of their ability at that particular time—if a child could do it better, they would.

If your child's speech is difficult to understand and your child is struggling to learn new speech sounds, contact your local SLP as soon as possible. It is always best to get some help and support.

**Top Tip Time** **Finessing speech sounds**

Look at the following list of commonly mispronounced sounds, find your child's specific speech-sound error, and follow the advice given.

**"P"**

"P" is often replaced with "b" or "d"—for instance, "pig" is spoken as "big" or "dig," or it may simply become "ig." At my clinic, I usually take a rectangular piece of paper and cut strips up the long side, not cutting the strips off completely. Hold the strips next to your mouth and say "p, p, p"—you will notice that the paper "jumps." Then hold it next to your child's mouth and encourage them to say "p, p, p." The jumping paper will motivate them to want to say the sound again. Once they can say "p," keep the paper by their mouth and say other words that start with "p" (for instance, "paper," "pea," "purse," and "pancake"). You could then encourage them to use minimal pairs, which are pairs of rhyming words using the incorrect and the target sound (for example, "pea"/"bee," "bow"/"dough," or "pig"/"dig").

## "B"

This is a lip sound and very similar to "p" and "m." Try using a straw to drink, which can improve all three of these sounds because this exercises the lips into a closed position. "B" is often replaced with "d," so encourage the "b" sound on its own, then use minimal pairs work (see above, under "P") to encourage your child to hear the difference between the rhyming words (examples are "bug"/"dug" and "boo"/"do").

## "M"

I often practice this with the help of some lip balm. Rub it on your child's lips and encourage them to rub their lips together and then say "mmm." Next, try replacing the "brum" noise of a motorbike with "mmm," and, eating chocolate, say "mmm" every time a piece goes in their mouth (I should be saying "delicious apple" but, honestly, chocolate will work better). Once they have got the sound right, try again and encourage them to say words beginning with "m" (for instance, "Mum," "moo," and "milk").

## "K"/"c"/"g"

Open your mouth, put your finger on your tongue so that your tongue tip stays in the base of your mouth and say "k, k, k." The same technique applies for "g." These sounds are often replaced with "t" and "d"—for instance, "car" becomes "tar," "gate" is said as "date," and "leg" becomes "led." You could also try minimal pairs—for example, "Kate"/"gate" and "key"/"tea." If the finger-on-your-tongue technique doesn't work, try to make that rather disgusting noise when you're trying to clear phlegm from your throat, which achieves closure of the back of the tongue against the roof of the mouth to make the sound. This should be in place by 3 years.

## "Qu"/"x"

"Qu" (as in "queen") is a blend of the consonants "k" and "w," and "x" (as in "exciting") is a "k" and "s" sound blended together. So, these sounds are blends, which are difficult to say before the age of 5. In order to say both sounds, a child would need to be able to say "k" first, then add the second consonant.

## "F"

The "f" sound is often replaced with a "b" sound, so "four" becomes "bour." To encourage your child to make this sound correctly, ask them to bite their bottom lip and blow out—like a rabbit's teeth. In fact, as a rabbit has no noise, I've taught my daughter to say "ff ff" when I say, "What does a rabbit say?," in preparation for the start of her trying to say "f" words later on. You could also try placing a piece of breakfast cereal on your child's bottom lip and encouraging them to remove it with their top teeth. This will encourage them to move their mouth into the correct mouth shape.

## "V"

This is a tricky sound—you might hear "TV" as "TD" or "van" as "ban." The "v" sound comes much later, at about 4½ years, so don't worry too much about it now—it's articulated in the same way as the "f" sound (see the previous section).

## "S"

This sound is often mistaken for "t" or "d," so "sun" is said as "dun." "S" is usually spoken correctly by 3½ years. Also, "s" can be lisped in three different ways.

1. A dentalized lisp, in which the child's tongue pops out between their teeth.
2. A lateral "s," which sounds like the Welsh "ll" sound (for example, "I want llome llaullagell [some sausages]").

3. A palatal "s." Say "y" and feel the middle of the tongue lift up toward the roof of your mouth. Keeping your tongue in that position, say "s"—that's what a palatal "s" sounds like.

Lisps are very common and, at 3 to 4 years, we don't worry massively about them so long as the child has an approximation of an "s" sound. A trick that I use to help children find the sound is to encourage them to say "t t t t t t" as fast as they can, so that the sound turns into an "s" sound. Try it. Play around with this technique before you introduce it to your child.

If you want to describe to your child how to say "s," say, "Put your tongue behind your teeth, bite, smile and blow out—'s s s s.'"

Be aware that it is unusual for air to come out of your child's nose when they say "s." If this happens, hold your child's nose and see what happens. Does a perfect sound come out? If so, you need to go and see an ear, nose, and throat specialist because this indicates a problem with the palate and needs further investigation. Otherwise, this speech-sound error is a placement problem and the usual tricks should work.

Use the tongue-behind-your-teeth technique for each of these lisps mentioned, but you may need some extra guidance for the lateral "s," which is particularly difficult to conquer. I would suggest you see an SLP who will try to achieve a good sound in the first session. Depending on this and the motivation of the child, the SLP may tell you to go away until the child notices or wants to change it. You'll have to consider this carefully. If you battle on with a sound that is very difficult to achieve, you run the risk of causing a lot of angst (rather like forcing a child to play a musical instrument) and making them less cooperative, which could affect your relationship with your child.

## "Sh"

This is commonly thought of as a tough sound to master. "Sh" is often replaced with "d" in the early stages and then, later on, "s," so "shoe" becomes "du" and then "sue," for example. Close your teeth, push your lips forward in a circle, and blow out. Encourage your child to do the same and put their finger by their lips so that their lips can reach for the finger when they are protruded. Once they've got it, go outside and say "shh" to any noise you hear! Seventy-five percent of 4-year-olds should say this sound correctly.

### "Ch"

This sound is often replaced with "t" or "d" and, later, with "ty" or "ts," so "chair" becomes "dair," "tyair" or "tsair." It is articulated in the same way as the "sh" sound (see above), so a child must try to achieve a "sh" sound first. Once they have, encourage them to put a little "t" and "sh" together. You might need a picture of a dripping faucet, to represent "t," and a mummy saying "shh" to a baby to help achieve this.

Start practicing this exercise when a child can speak in short sentences or if they aren't saying the "ch" sound correctly by approximately age 4.

### "J"

The "j" sound comes as a pair with the "ch" sound, so once your child has cracked "ch," "j" should follow naturally at about 4½ years.

### "L"

A child will usually replace this sound with "w," so "lemon" becomes "wemon," for instance. The easiest way for a child to see the correct position for their tongue is in a mirror, so encourage your child to lift their tongue up onto the ridge behind their top front teeth, then say "l," as they look at the shape both their and your mouths are making in the mirror.

Start practicing this if a child isn't saying it correctly by approximately 4 years of age.

## "Th"

This sound will usually be replaced with "f," so "three" becomes "free." To produce the sound, encourage your child to bite their tongue and blow out—try it yourself. Once they have mastered this, encourage them to say "thin," "the," "thing," and other words beginning with "th."

Start practicing this exercise if your child isn't saying it correctly by approximately 6 years. If your child is struggling with this sound now, please don't worry.

## "R"

This is quite a difficult sound to explain to a child. Most children replace "r" with "w." The main difference between the two sounds is the position of the tongue. Try it. I usually encourage a child to practice saying the two sounds after each other so they can hear that they are saying "w" for both sounds. If you hear two "w" sounds, you will have to teach your child how to say "r" by telling them to lift their tongue tip up toward the roof of their mouth, then smile and blow out for an "r" sound and curl their lips into a circle for the "w" sound. Once this is achieved, tell them to say a vowel and then "r"—for example, "eeer" or "aaaar," so they can feel their tongue moving upward after the vowel. Try this for a couple of days, then try adding the same vowel to the end of the "word," too—for example, "eeereee" or "aaaraa."

Start practicing this exercise if your child isn't saying this sound correctly by approximately 6 years and, until then, don't worry about it.

## Blends

The following consonant blends might be tricky for a child of a young age to achieve.

- "S" blends: "sn," "sm," "sl," "sw," "sk," "st," "squ"
- "L" blends: "fl," "cl," "sl," "gl," "pl," "bl"
- "R" blends: "cr," "fr," "dr," "tr," "gr," "br," "pr"

It's difficult for children to blend two consonant sounds together. Usually, a child will drop one of the sounds or change the blend altogether, so "snake" becomes "nake," "clock" is said as "cock," "blue" becomes "bue," "train" becomes "dain," and "princess" is said as "bincess." So you might hear, "A pider [spider] followed me to the twings [swings] and down the side [slide]."

Before you practice these blends with your child, you must ensure that they are able to say each consonant in the blend individually. So, if your child can say "f" and "l" clearly, they're ready to try to say "flower." Encourage them to listen to each sound. For instance, you might say, "Let's say the sounds for train—'tr-ai-n.' Can you hear 'tr'? It's a 't' and an 'r' together. Let's say it: 't' then 'r' is 'tr tr tr.'" Then add the rest of the word—"tr-ain." Ensure you don't say "tuh" and "ruh," because the word "train" does not sound like "tuh-ruh-ain." (See my explanation about Tracey's daughter Minnie, pages 142–43.)

It is always a good idea to practice these as minimal pairs—for example, "peas"/"please," "gate"/"great," and "tick"/"stick."

Start practicing these sounds if your child isn't saying them correctly by approximately six years—until then, don't worry about it.

I have left out "t" and "d" purposely as it is unusual not to be able to say these sounds. If your child can't say these sounds by the age of 3, I would suggest they see an SLP for some guidance. Difficulty saying them is associated with dummy sucking—if this is the case, ditch the dummy as soon as possible.

It might just take a few simple sound games to master these sounds, but very often it takes longer. If this is the case, you will need to go back to the eight-stage process on pages 145–51. Just be patient. I often say to worried parents that very few 7- or 8-year-olds don't speak clearly—most children have sorted out their speech-sound mistakes by this age.

Be aware of the sounds your child can and can't say and try to encourage them in a fun and motivating way, so you don't make them feel self-conscious or negative about the way they speak. Seek help if you are worried. Generally, SLPs worry more about language problems than speech-sound problems (this, of course, depends on the severity of the speech-sound error).

It's when children start chatting away, telling made-up stories, that you may begin to notice that they are getting certain sounds or words a bit wrong. They might say "foots" for "feet" or "goed" instead of "went," because they're still trying to work out how language works and master the rules behind it. You might still have words that are mispronounced, such as "busgeti" (spaghetti), "wimmin" (swimming), and "aminal" (animal)—which you'll "ploberly" find totally endearing. Speech sounds can be tricky, but generally SLP's are more concerned that a child is understanding and has a means to express themself rather than worrying too much about how pretty the word sounds. Before very long, your child will become a little parrot copying everything you say. This is when you and your partner will have to become that parenting cliché and spell out the words you don't want your child to copy from you. (For example, "How was your day, dear?" "Darling, it was C-R-A-P! Please take him to the P-A-R-K so I can have a glass of wine.")

Chapter 8

# What to do when . . .
# your child isn't speaking
# in sentences

Most children go through a "big boom" stage—the explosion of single-word expansion, and single words into short phrases. In fact, there might come a time where your child's vocabulary could *double* in the period of just a few months. And, by the end of their fourth year, some children will know 500 to 600 words and some could know as many as 1,000—that's a 500 percent increase from the average of 100 to 200 or so words that is expected at 2 years of age. At some point between their second and third year, some parents see their child effortlessly learn as many as 9 or 10 new words a day! How easy it is for some! And how near on impossible it seems for others . . .

Let's remind ourselves just why language is so important. You need language for remembering ("Why is Daddy putting me to bed tonight? Oh yes, because Mummy went to the movies"), thinking and reasoning ("Why won't that shape fit into that hole?" or "Why has my daddy got to go to work?"), for self-control ("I'm not allowed to climb the stairs so I won't," or in my case, "Don't have another chocolate cookie"!), and planning ("Shall we go swimming or to the swings today?"). We also need language for dealing with emotions and worries, making friends, and, of course, communicating.

In this chapter, we've reached the point where a child is using short phrases and simple sentences, so we'll be covering three key areas.

- **Concepts:** hot, cold, clean, dirty, long, short, fat, thin
- **Grammar:** helping your child develop the intricacies of their word and sentence structure to make longer and more complex sentences ("dog bark" might change to "the dog is barking") and to use more advanced grammar such as correct word endings and appropriate pronouns ("me go" becomes "I'm going"), plurals (cats, horses)
- **Memory:** This evolving skill is crucial for further language development, and I'll give you tips to give that gray matter a boost!

Once your little one has begun to master and combine these three core elements, you'll notice that they will suddenly want to start telling *you* stories. So, we'll also learn about narrative skills and look at how you can create many elaborate tales to tell.

So, all of the Top Tip Times in this chapter are geared around working toward achieving these impressive milestones. Won't it be lovely to sit back and have your little one tell *you* a story?


## CONCEPTS

Let's consider the concept of a "tree." Although there's an extraordinary array of different types of tree in the world (different sizes, shapes, colors, textures, fruits, seasonal changes, life spans, and so on), they all fall under the single category of "tree." So, your child may be able to say the word *tree* if they see an oak, for example, but not have a sense of the concept of what a tree is. But as their ability to think develops, they will become interested in finding out about a tree —or what the concept of a tree is. They'll begin to notice the features that make this oak a tree and not a plant, a flower, or a piece of wood. Therefore, the true definition of a concept is an idea, thought, or notion—a mental category that helps us to classify particular objects or events that share a set of common features or attributes.

At about the age of 2 to 2½ years, some children begin to understand size concepts, such as "big" and "little," and the quantity concepts, such as "all" or "none." Then, at about 2½ to 3 years, there is often a massive expansion of the understanding of more complex concepts—such as those of location (for example, in/on/under) and time (today/tomorrow).

Alongside this expansive interest in things, your child might start to ask a barrage of questions—you will hear "What?" and "Who?," and a bit later, "Where?," "When?," and "Why?" will be added to the list (at which point, parents may begin struggling to provide the answers). After all, why is a tree not a plant? For those of us who aren't botanists or even gardeners, the answer isn't always obvious. Our daily language is full of concepts, and we have to teach our little ones to understand them and to use them. In the following, we look at ideas for how to do this.

## Teaching your child general concepts

Remember that a child must have a good understanding of a concept before using it expressively. Therefore, there are two stages to learning any new concept—first, helping your little one to understand the word and, second, encouraging them to use it.

The concepts likely to catch the eyes—and the imaginations—of children of this age are the more distinctive/obvious ones. Understanding the more subtle concepts comes later. So, "fat" is likely to come before "thin," "large" before "small," "tall" before "short," and so on. I laughed and cringed when Tracey told me when she knew that Minnie had obviously grasped the "fat" concept; they were shopping in the supermarket and wheeled their cart past a couple, when Minnie said very clearly, "That was a fat man, wasn't it?" Tracey zoomed away as quickly as she could and then explained to Minnie that it wasn't kind to say things like that about someone's appearance.

You might have to develop a thick skin as your child begins describing the world around them using these new concepts without a care for social etiquette, but I can assure you that you'll probably laugh more than you'll blush. And, of course, the most embarrassing gaffes will become part of your child's oral history, just like those first words!

The following are examples of the concepts to try to incorporate into your daily life and during your 10 minutes of Special Time while playing. Following them are some Top Tip Time games that will help you to practice. The goal is to get your child familiar with the label of a word, and then understand the concept of it and the context in which to use it. Here are the key concepts.

- On/Off
- Same/Different
- Happy/Sad
- Full/Empty
- Loud/Quiet
- Old/Young
- Up/Down
- More/Less
- Top/Bottom
- Big/Little
- All/None
- Front/Back
- Old/New
- Long/Short
- Hard/Soft
- Over/Under
- Hot/Cold

- Smooth/Rough
- Forward/Backward
- Above/Below

**Top Tip Time** **Teaching your little one concepts**

Remember—language develops through play, so be aware of what your child loves to play with and what they are motivated by so that you can find as many opportunities as possible to develop their use of concepts as they toddle about.

- Mealtimes give you a great opportunity to teach concepts. First, name all the food to extend your child's vocabulary, then talk about the concepts. Fish fingers are "rough," but the fish in the middle is "smooth." That yogurt is "cold" because it has been in the refrigerator. By doing this you are helping your child to understand concepts by talking about the object and thinking about how it fits into their world.

- Share books, and if the illustrations lend themselves to teaching a variety of concepts (for example, big/little, happy/sad, long/short), point them out. Believe it or not, *Thomas the Tank Engine* books are really good for teaching emotional concepts—the trains have the most exaggerated facial expressions, which are great!

- You can buy "opposites books" that have concepts in them. We have a book called *Spot's Opposites* by Eric Hill at my clinic. I also like *The Baby's Catalogue* by Janet and Allan Ahlberg, which is full of everyday pictures of family life and is good for learning concepts. There is a page of garden objects, a family page, a breakfast page, etc. The book contains pictures of things to describe as soft, hard, hot, cold, prickly, smooth, big, little, and so on.

- Collect from around your house objects that are big and little, or the same and different, or soft and hard. Talk about these objects with your child.

- Play the game I Spy, using attributes to describe the chosen object—for example, "I spy something that is soft."

- Play the game I Went to the Store and Bought . . . When you take turns to add something new to the end of the list, introduce a concept. For example, you could say, "I went to the store and bought a big cake," and your child says, "I went to the store and bought a big cake and a new hat," and so on. Also try, "I went to the zoo and saw a tall giraffe," then "I went to the zoo and saw a tall giraffe and a thin snake."

- Try drawing, painting, or molding with Play-Doh things that are opposites—for example, long and short snakes, big and little balls, fat and thin cats, high and low mountains—and talking about them. Ask your child to explain them to another adult.

- This age group loves "container play"—filling and dumping objects into containers, handbags, baskets, etc. Give your child a pile of objects that are hard/soft, rough/smooth, heavy/light, and so on, to put into containers.

- Children of this age often have a strong desire to dress themselves and be independent, so let your child choose their clothes and describe the clothes as they put them on (for instance, "Oh, you've found something with long sleeves/a heavy sweater/a pretty shirt").

- Engage in symbolic play and act out household activities with a running commentary involving concepts—for example, "We're wiping the dirty table—now it's clean," or "We're vacuuming the soft carpet and then the hard wood." Talk to your toddler about the activity as they help to tidy the house—you can't go wrong with this one!

- Your child should also be able to imitate vertical strokes on paper, so say "down" as the brush goes down and encourage them to say "up" as the brush goes up. You could try painting "fast" or "slow" or with "thin" or "thick" stripes.

- Get your child to tear up some paper, then talk about "big" pieces and "small" pieces. They'll love pasting them down, too.

- Lastly, try categorizing a range of objects in play. For example, "Let's put all the noisy farm animals/all the summer clothes together," and "Let's tidy all the big books into this box and all the small puzzles onto the tray."

## COMPARATIVES AND SUPERLATIVES (–ER AND –EST)

Once your child has grasped some of the concepts listed previously, why not use these words to compare and contrast things with each other? So, when your child can say "big tractor," show them that we can be even more specific about its size and explain that even though this tractor is big, that one is even bigger, but the one over there is the biggest. What excitement that'll bring on!

**Top Tip Time** Bigger, biggest, and best!

- Line up a range of objects in order of size. Size differences are visual and are therefore easier to grasp. Jumble them up and line them up again. Ask which is the biggest, then go along the line and say, "This car is bigger than that car, this car is bigger than that car, and this one is the biggest." Make sure your child understands the words *bigger* and *biggest*.

- Again, use food at mealtimes to talk about size comparisons. First, use two objects—for example, "I have a big cup, but your cup is bigger," "This potato is big, but that one is bigger," or "Your hands are big, but my hands are bigger." When you say the word "bigger," sign it to emphasize the size by stretching your hands apart. Once you think your child understands this concept, try three objects to go through the same format—for instance, "My cup is big, your cup is bigger, but this cup is the biggest!"

Go through the same format with other tangible objects. For instance, use the comparatives and superlatives as you load the washing machine using sock length, smelliness, or dirtiness—this should appeal to a little one's sense of humor! Make sure you use only regular forms at this stage (which are those ending in the regular –er and –est ending—for instance, hot/hotter/hottest, happy/happier/happiest, quiet/quieter/quietest and soft/softer/softest).

Later, you will find that your child generalizes this pattern and applies it erroneously to irregular forms, so she'll use "badder" rather than "worse" or "worst"; "good," "gooder," and "good-est" rather than "good," "better," and "best"; and "beautiful," "beautifuler," and "beautifulest" rather than "more beautiful" or "most beautiful." There are many other irregular patterns, so you will have to sensitively model the correct form back in a positive way. When your child says, "This is my bestest toy," you can reply, "That's right. It's your best toy."

## TEACHING YOUR CHILD PREPOSITIONS

Prepositions are words (or spatial concepts) that describe a location, such as "in," "on," "under," "in front," "behind," and so on. First, your child will learn to understand these words and then begin to use them. The first prepositions children tend to understand are "in," "on," and "under," and as soon as they understand them, they learn to say them.

So, before embarking on prepositions, make sure your child can say two-word sentences and understand three-word sentences. Start with putting a preposition into a few-word sentence—for example, "It's under the blanket."

Prepositions are crucial for your child to learn, as they will help them to expand their sentence length, enable them to answer a "where" question, and retell a story or an event in greater detail. Let's think about some Top Tip Time games that will help your child to learn prepositions.

**Top Tip Time** **Getting into space, man!**

In order of difficulty, what follows is a list of the prepositions your child will master.

- In/Out
- On
- Up/Down

- Under
- Behind
- In Front of
- On Top of
- At the Bottom of
- Over
- Near/Next to
- Beside
- Between

The games that follow are listed in order of difficulty, so progress through them in sequence (as much as possible). They involve your child physically putting themself into a position, then putting a toy or an object into a position, and, last, using the word without any visual information to help them.

1. Begin with a physical demonstration, like standing ON the rug or sitting UNDER the table—say what you are doing. Then have your child perform the same actions while you describe what they do. This will help them understand the prepositions. Why not take photos so that you can talk about them later?

   To make this game more fun, play hide-and-seek— leave the room and tell your child to "Hide UNDER the cushions!" Or make up an obstacle course out of furniture, enabling you both to climb over, under, on top, beside, and between things.

2. There are a number of nursery rhymes that use prepositions (see the list that follows). Sing these and act out the prepositions, then talk about them.

   » "Ring Around the Rosie" (we all fall down)
   » "The Hokey Pokey" (in/out)
   » "Roly Poly, Roly Poly, Up Up Up" (up/down)

» "Jack and Jill" (up/down)

» "Hey Diddle Diddle" (over)

3. Hide a small toy in, on, or under a box and direct your child to find it, telling them that it is "in the box," "under the box," and so on. Model the words for them so they learn their meaning.

4. Try to incorporate prepositions into your daily routine. For instance:

» When tidying up, ask your child to put things in specific places ("Put your pajamas under your pillow," "Put bunny on the chair").

» When you're loading the washing machine, say, "Put your pants in the machine."

» When wiping the table, say, "Here's the cloth, wipe under your plate."

» When in the bath, say, "Wash in your ears, under your chin, next to your belly button."

5. Read books that have prepositions, such as *Where's Spot?* and *We're Going on a Bear Hunt* (in which the repetitive line is "We can't go over it, we can't go under it . . .").

6. Once you feel your child is able to understand these concepts, move on to tabletop activities. Draw pictures of people or animals in, on, under, in front of, and behind things. Also, cut out pictures from magazines of people in, on, under, in front of, and behind things.

7. Ask your child to help you with some basic cooking. Use this opportunity to talk about what is going "in" the mixing bowl, what is "on" the table, and where items are (for instance, "The spoon is *under* the lid").

# MASTERING SIMPLE USE OF GRAMMAR

The introduction of grammar will come after your child's language boom, so that's after a child has started using two key words in a sentence (see Top Tips on how to encourage two-word sentences). It is said that children need to understand 200 to 250 words before they understand grammar, and should be able to say the same number of words before spoken grammar appears.

Picking up grammar isn't easy. Grammatically, English is brutal, as there are so many irregularities. And it's irrational to think of a tiny tot's brain absorbing all these grammatical rules without even flinching. Even more incredible is the fact that children don't just know the rules; they truly understand their logic. In a famous experiment by the world-leading psycholinguist Jean Berko Gleason in 1958, children were presented with a fantasy creature rather like a bird and were told it was a "wug"—an invented word—and then shown a second wug. The English-speaking children invariably said "two wugs," demonstrating that they had learned the grammatical rule of plurals and could transfer this knowledge to a completely new word.

The mistakes children make also show us how deep their understanding of grammar is and how they apply it. "We swimmed" is a great example of a child applying a perfectly logical rule to the past tense of the English language; it just happens that this is one of our many irregular verbs. This overgeneralization of the rule persists until the child has sorted out the instances in which the general rules apply and those in which they are overruled by the irregular verb. Amazingly, many children are likely to have grasped most of these irregularities by the age of 3½ to 4 years. Truly amazing.

## How does grammar develop?

You may want to know a bit more about the order in which grammatical rules are picked up and when (and do a bit of revision yourself on possessive pronouns and the like—most of us have no idea what all these conjugations are called; our brain just automatically arranges the grammar correctly for us). In his book *A First Language* (1973), the researcher Roger Brown outlined the developmental stages in grammar. This model is still used by SLPs today to predict the progressive path that expressive language development usually takes.

### Stage 1 (at about 2 years)

A child learns to put two words together. They should have just about conquered this at the age of 2.

### Stage 2 (roughly between 2 and 3 years)

A child will learn to

- use the possessive "s," so phrases like "man's book" appear, and begin to use their name when talking about themself,
- introduce pronouns, such as "my," "mine," "you," "me" and "he" and "she,"
- add "-ing" to the end of a verb ("I am runn*ing*"),
- use plurals ("one banana, two bananas"),
- use negatives ("no," "not," "can't"),
- raise their intonation for a question, and
- begin to use the past tense.

### Stage 3 (roughly between 3 and 3½ years)

A child will learn to

- inconsistently use the present tense auxiliaries "can" and "will"—for example, "I can swim" or "I will come," and
- overgeneralize the past tense—for example, "goed" instead of "went" or "writed" instead of "wrote."

The Top Tip Time games that follow focus on the areas of grammar that should have been mastered by the time a child reaches about 3 to 3½ years of age.

**Top Tip Time** **Adding "-ing" to the end of a verb**

Here are some regular verbs to start you off: play, kick, jump, cry, wash, walk, brush, push, paint, cook, dance.

- Take pictures of your child or someone else doing these actions and collate them into a slideshow. Ask your child, "What is happenING?" Remind them to listen to the question, particularly listening to the "–ing" ending. Make sure they use a matching "–ing" ending in response to the question—for instance, "The girl is jumping," or "Mummy is dancing." Children often start by saying "girl running" and miss out the "is," but this is fine and you can simply model the correct phrase by saying, "Yes, well done, the girl is running." Print out your photos and make up some flash cards to practice with.

- Play charades. Take turns acting out an action, then guess the action using the "–ing" form. Afterward, you can talk about the game in the past tense to get your child thinking about the next phase, saying, for instance, "First you jumped and then you danced."

**Top Tip Time** **Plurals**

When we want to signify that there is more than one of something, we make it plural by adding an "s" to the end of a word (for instance, "one cat, three cats"). However, some words are irregular and don't follow this rule. If your child is having difficulty with this, help by first practicing regular plurals where you simply add "s."

- If your child leaves the "s" off the word—by asking for "raisin for Erin," for instance—only give one raisin, then model, "Erin wants raisinSSSSS. Raisins for Erin." Or if your child says, "Dan shoe on," put on one shoe and look puzzled. Model the phrase again, "Dan shoesssss on," before putting the second one on.

- Draw some pictures of objects. On one page, put one object, and on the other put many (one flower and three flowers or one pig and two pigs, for instance). Talk through the pictures with your child, emphasizing the "s" ending on the plurals.

- Play I Spy, choosing plural objects to spy. For instance, you might pick "booksssssssss" if there are lots of them in the room.

- When your child is talking, remind them of plurals by saying things like, "Was there one chip on your plate or lots?," and when they say "lots," remind them that they need to say "chipssssss."

- Try finding groups of objects to talk about. For instance, separate one pea from a group of peas on a dinner plate and say, "One pea, lots of peas." This works with everything from blocks to animals.

- Think of things that come in pairs (socks, shoes, Noah's ark animals). Practice the singular and plural forms for each word—for example, "glove" and "gloves."

- When your child has mastered regular plurals, introduce the irregular plurals (for example, mouse/mice, sheep/sheep, fish/fish, child/children, foot/feet) using the methods above.

**Top Tip Time** **Negatives**

During the terrible twos, "no" and "don't" tend to become rather popular negatives! You'll hear things like "no juice" and "no want bedtime." Use the following tips to help your child understand negatives.

- Draw pictures of three people—the first two wearing hats but not the third. Say, "Hat, hat, no hat." Shake your head to make it more understandable. Try this again using faces and a nose ("Nose, nose, no nose"). Encourage your child to join in.

- At the end of a meal, offer "More?" If they say no, say, "No more."

- Open the refrigerator and play the following game: "I like yogurt but I don't like mustard. I like butter but I don't like tomato sauce." Look at the toy section in a catalog and say, "I like Elmo but I don't like Oscar the Grouch," and so on.

At about 2½ to 3 years, the "not," "none" and "nobody" words appear. For example, a child might say, "Do you want more or not?" Use the tips below to encourage this development.

- Look through picture books and take opportunities to use these words. For instance, you might say, "Crocodile is hiding under the bed," then turn the page and say, "Monkey is not hiding under the bed, monkey is in the wardrobe. Who is hiding under the table? Nobody is hiding under the table."

- The most common use for the word *none* is in answer to the question "Can I have a cookie?"—"No, there are none left!" Emphasize the word *none* as your child absorbs the impact of the concept of an empty cookie jar!

**Top Tip Time** **Pronouns**

Essentially, pronouns relate to how we refer to ourselves and others. Pronouns tend to emerge anywhere between 19 and 24 months. Your child's grasp of pronouns will probably begin when they start talking about themself in the third person—for instance, "Anabelle drink." This is rather more charming than what comes next—*mine*, a word you are likely to hear all too frequently (usually accompanied by a toy clutched in a fist and a frowning face!). At around 2 to 2½ years, this develops into "my," "me," and "you," so you'll probably begin hearing, "My can do it!," "Me do it!," and then, "I," "mine," and "yours."

Later, at about 30 months, your child could be able to distinguish between a boy and a girl and begin using "he," "she," and "they," if this is what you'd like to teach them. Children often become muddled between "he" and "she"—you might hear your child say "that one" instead!

Use the following ideas to help your child practice pronouns.

- Play at dealing cards, saying, "One for me and one for you . . ."
- When you are sorting clothes, say, "Daddy's shirt," "your pants," and so on, and encourage your toddler to pick something up and say, "my jacket," "your socks."

- Take photos of yourself and your child doing things and discuss these with them, saying, "I am swimming," and so on. Take their hand and encourage them to point at themself when they say "I." Then show them a picture of you doing something and take their hand and point to yourself and say, "You are drinking."

Before a child can use pronouns, we have to be certain that they know the difference between "boy," "girl," and any other options. So, you can ask, "Is Daddy a boy or a girl?" And you can adapt these questions, depending on how you identify and want to teach gender to your child. Start practicing "he," "she," and "they," using the following tips.

- Collect old family photos or cut out pictures from magazines of boys, girls, and groups of people together. Say corresponding things, such as, "What is *she* doing?" or "*She* is wearing a hat." Reverse roles, so your little one has to ask the questions using the correct pronouns.

- Use Playmobil or Duplo characters to make up a simple story; for instance, make the characters play hide-and-seek. Retell the story using pronouns ("He was hiding in the car," "They were under the bed," and so on).

- Talk about everyday experiences as they happen ("He is eating," or "They are happy").

Later, try "his," "hers," and "theirs," which is expected at around 3½ years.

- Use pictures of a boy, a girl, and a group and select some real food. Ask your child to close their eyes and then allocate a different piece of food to the boy and girl. When they open their eyes ask, "What's for *her* dinner?" Encourage them to respond with a pronoun in a full sentence (you may have to model the sentence type you want several times first), such as "*Her* dinner is fish." Reverse the roles.

## Auxiliaries

Omitting auxiliaries like "can" and "will" is quite common from the age of 2. When these words are left out, the meaning of the sentence usually remains intact. (I suppose the sentence is grammatically correct and therefore just sounds more grown-up and "prettier" when the auxiliaries are used.)

The earliest form of auxiliary you'll notice your child using will probably be "is" and "am"—basically, the verb "to be."

### Is

People usually say "he's" rather than "he is," but it is easier to hear the latter form and therefore we tend to practice this and wait for a child to naturally shorten it. So, you would model "he is running" or "my sock is wet" and over time, your child will shorten these sentences to "he's running" and "my sock's wet."

### Am

Here are some examples of a child missing "am" out of a sentence: "I in sandpit," "I cold," and "I upset and cry." Model the correct sentence using "I am," which they'll shorten to "I'm" over time.

### Have

Again, we usually say, "I've drawn a picture," rather than "I have drawn a picture," so if you hear your child say, "I drawn a picture," model the correct sentence back using "have."

## VERBAL REASONING

You'll find it easier to reason with your little one as their language and understanding reach a higher level and they understand sentences along the lines of, "If you don't put your puzzle away, I'll call Louise's mum and tell her not to come and play."

Of course, the result is that parenting can feel rather like a high-level negotiating role at the United Nations, but there is something thrilling about being able to reason with your child, and their reasoning back. They are becoming a little person, with their own logic and ideas (even if their logic is sometimes a little out of left field!).

**Top Tip Time** **Possessives**

Children can get terribly confused between plurals and the possessive "s" (for instance, "the ladies" or "the lady's house") so we need to encourage them to think about the words carefully.

- Use real objects (clothes are good) to practice using possessives. Say, "Whose sock is this? It's Daddy's," or "Whose book is this? It's Fabian's."

- When you are going out, get your child to sort out the clothing, saying, "That's Freddie's coat/Tom's shoe/Daddy's glasses," and so on.

- Take photos of your child with belongings, and discuss the pictures with them, saying, "It's Ella's tractor," and so on.

- Cut out pictures of toys from a catalog and gather pictures of your child and people they know. Stick them into a book, with the picture of a person on the left-hand page, and an object on the opposite page. Then look through the book with your tiny tot, modeling "Adam's Jeep," "Lola's fairy wings," and so on.

---

## HOW WILL YOUR CHILD'S GRAMMAR DEVELOP?

At about age 2, a child will still employ overextension, using the same word to refer to a number of different objects. A child at this age also uses underextension (the opposite of overextension). For example, a child may only call black Labradors—and no other dogs—"dog," or call their own boots "boots," calling other boots "that" or "shoes." But, over time, this will change and your child will even learn to request clarification.

---

## MEMORY

It's only natural to focus on the parts of language you can hear—the talking—and dismiss the aspects of language development that aren't so apparent, such as concentration, memory, and understanding. But you need to be able to focus, remember, and understand words before you can say them. So, in this section, we will think about memory and its importance in the language-development process.

There are three types of memory that are crucial for language development. These are long-term memory (LTM), short-term memory (STM), and working memory (WM). To explain this, I can use the example of a telephone conversation I had with my mum to arrange what to do on Mother's Day.

When my mum mentioned Mother's Day, my long-term memory enabled me to remember our plan from last year—to have a family lunch. It was a disaster. All the children were tired (it was their nap time) so they fussed throughout the meal. Because my mother and I could remember this, we could describe and explain why we shouldn't do the same this year. During the discussion, as each sentence was being spoken, it was processed and retained momentarily in our working memory, but then forgotten (meaning that, after the call, I wouldn't have been able to retell the conversation word for word). The finer details of times and plans were stored in my short-term memory for a brief period of time. Once the day was over, because the details were not rehearsed over and over again after the event, they weren't stored in my long-term memory, so they have been forgotten.

Your memory systems work together so that what is said can be immediately processed by the working memory, taken into your short-term memory, and then, when the information is stored and understood, it will either be linked with existing knowledge in the long-term memory or forgotten. This is how our children learn everything from new words and sentence structure to what their routine is at breakfast and how they play with building blocks.

There's nothing more frustrating than forgetting a name when you see someone or forgetting a word you want to use in the heat of the moment, so start training your child's memory now!

## MEMORY NORMS

- At about 18 months, a child should be able to echo or repeat the last word or the most predominant word in a sentence.

- At about 2 years, a child should have a working memory (also known as auditory memory, as they are remembering what they have heard) of two objects.

- At about 2 to 2½ years, a child can sequence two pieces of information in order, so they should remember two key elements in a longer command (for instance, "Pick up the brush and give it to Daddy").

- At about 3 to 4 years, a child should remember three key objects.

# WHY IS A GOOD WORKING MEMORY SO IMPORTANT?

Experts say that if you test working memory in preschool, you can predict academic success three years later. So, a good working memory is the key to successful learning and goes hand-in-hand with speech and language development, and a good verbal working memory can be an indicator of intelligence.

**Top Tip Time**  **Memory Boosters**

A child's memory is assisted massively by their ability to sit still and listen—a seemingly impossible feat for some little ones. So, ensure your child has excellent listening skills (see tips on improving listening skills, pages 60–63) so they can listen for language.

- Learning to sing the words to your child's favorite song is a great test for their memory and something that they will love to do. Encourage them by providing actions or props to help them visualize the words in the song (for example, the actions in the song "Baby Shark"). When a word or a message is attached to a tune, you can remember it more easily, so don't just stop at singing songs—sing a message, too! If you feel uncomfortable singing, just make your voice as singsongy or as rhythmical as possible so that your child can tune in to it and remember it more easily.

- Ask your little one to remember a message and deliver it to someone in a different room (for instance, "Can you ask Louis if he would like a snack?" or "Tell Daddy Mummy wants a drink").

- Take a set of musical instruments. Play one shake of the tambourine, followed by a ting on the triangle and one clap of the hands—see if your child can copy the sequence. Change the sequence.

- Encourage your child to remember an item of food from the shopping list as you go around the supermarket. Can she remember two, then three, and maybe even four things that you need to buy?

- Try the following simple repetition memory games.
  - » **Noises:** Do one noise first and get your child to copy, then add another to make two noises, then another to make three. Ask your child to copy you in sequence.
  - » **Words:** Place some pictures of objects that fall within one category (for instance, food, toys, or vehicles) on the floor facing upward. Encourage your child to remember, then repeat, then put a range of pictures either into a mailbox or into a puppet's mouth, saying "Give the puppet the car/bus/train."
  - » **Sentences:** Give your child an instruction. Encourage them to say it out aloud before they carry it out (for instance, "Rub your tummy" or "Touch your nose and jump").
- Play pairs with some cards and encourage your child to remember where a particular card is when it is placed upside down on a table.
- Hide objects around the room, then have a treasure hunt to find them. Or encourage your child to hide an object, then tell you where to find it.
- Place five or so objects on the table, take one away and ask your child to name the object that has disappeared.
- Assemble a few groups of objects and pictures and sort them into categories. Mix them all up again and see if your child can remember which item fits into a particular category.
- Your child will enjoy listening to familiar stories, so leave a key word out and see if they can fill it in. The next step might be to purposefully say the wrong thing to see if they notice and correct you. You could also encourage them to stay tuned in by telling them, "Every time I say 'lion,' why don't you roar like a lion?"
- Read a story to your child and encourage them to repeat it back (for more information see the following, Telling Stories).

> ## VERY ACTIVE BRAIN ALERT!
>
> The brain of a 3-year-old is two and a half times more active than an adult's. Forming all those neural pathways is a time-consuming task!

## TELLING STORIES

So, now your child's vocabulary is increasing, their memory is improving, and they are beginning to master concepts and grammar. And, when all these things start to click, children also begin to talk about absent objects to start a conversation. In other words, they move away from only referring to the here and now and their imaginations begin to run riot.

Here's a story my daughter tried to tell me.

Jess: "Granny hat."

Me: "Yes, Granny's hat blew away in the wind."

Jess: "Granny gone."

Me: "Yes, Granny ran after it!"

Your child will also talk about things that have happened during the day. With some prompting, they might be able to sequence things into a simple story—for example, "Me go outside." "And what did you do outside?" "Collect bugs." By about age 3, they might be able to tell a simple made-up story based on their own experiences or books they've read. They'll probably leave out lots of detail and rely on the listener to ask questions or interpret a meaning from the odd sentence or two (for example, "Max dressing up," after reading *Where the Wild Things Are*, or "Balloon in tree. Stuck," when, a few days before, her balloon had become stuck in a tree).

That's why narrative skills (being able to sequence a chain of events into a pattern so that they have some kind of significance) are a good indicator of how a child thinks and demonstrate their understanding of the experiences they have encountered.

If you want to boost your child's narrative skills, see the following Top Tips. Hearing your tiny talker's take on the day's events is certainly a great motivator. A child's observations and quirky eye for detail never fail to be entertaining.

**Top Tip Time** **Telling a story**

First of all, your child must listen to you retell stories over and over again, and learn a framework, to be able to retell their story. Try these ideas.

- The easiest way to achieve this is retelling things that you've done using the "first, then, and last" model. For instance, "First you sat in the dentist's chair, then you opened your mouth, and last you got a sticker." Or try using the same format to explain how to make a piece of toast, how to get dressed, and what happened when you went shopping.

- You can show your child a familiar photo and talk about it. Who is in it? Where were you? When was it? What happened next? Help them to answer these questions, then retell the story—for instance, "Mummy and Frankie went to the beach on my birthday. Then we built a big sandcastle and then the ocean washed it away."

- You can also make up stories about toys or people you know using the "first, then, and last" framework. Try to act them out. Words are much easier to learn when they are brought to life.

- Try using a talking teddy—you take teddy out on an event with you and retell what teddy did once it has happened. This technique is very popular in nurseries and schools.

- Try giving your child two objects, then make up a story. For example, for a dolly and a box, "Dolly said, 'I'm tired,' so she made a bed in a box and then went straight to sleep."

- Act out familiar stories such as *Rosie's Walk*, *Who Sank the Boat?*, *The Gruffalo*, *Five Minutes' Peace*, and *We're Going on a Bear Hunt*—my nephew loves this game.

- Cook together and think about the sequence of events that occurred as you gobble up your culinary delights. For instance, you could say, "First we measured the butter and flour, then we mixed them up with the egg, then we put it into the cake tin, and last, it was ready!"

- Fuzzy felts or misfits games are quite good for telling stories, or you can buy jigsaw puzzles that enable you to tell a story (all the pieces fit together so that you can put random pictures together).

- Read a familiar story and, before you turn the page, ask, "What happens next?" or "What happens at the end?"

- Color photocopy a favorite book (or I tend to buy a second copy of a classic book from a thrift shop) and cut out the pictures of the most significant events in the story. Then read the full book and ask your child to put the cut-up pictures into the story sequence.

## Make a story sack

The idea of story sacks was first created by Neil Griffiths, an ex-head-teacher-turned-children's writer, in 1997 (see storysack.com for more information). You read a story, then find objects that can help to bring the story to life (a teddy that resembles a character, props that can be used to represent scenery, noises or settings, and so on) and put them all in a bag. This is the ultimate visual support—by finding the real objects to talk about and learn about, your child can try to retell the story to you. Using this game is a lovely way to encourage your little one to tell stories, then listen to her imagination run wild. Try to nurture and develop this skill as much as you possibly can. It's something you can try yourself at home. I have just made a story sack for our clinic using the story *Handa's Surprise* by Eileen Browne. Into the sack went a doll, a basket, some fruit, and some animals, and it was good to go.

# Is your child telling stories?

Somewhere between the ages of about 2½ and 4 years, a child might begin to listen to stories with increasing attention, and soon after, they'll be able to sit and listen to a story for about 15 minutes. They will also be able to retell a short story, managing to describe the story setting, the basic sequence of events, and the central characters. The same information may be repeated and they may fixate on a particular part of the story, adding increasing information about it (which may or may not have been part of the original story!). They may then lose track of the plot altogether.

## FIVE ADDITIONAL WAYS TO PROMOTE CHILDREN'S CHATTER . . . ON A DAY OUT

1. **Simon Says:** Give your child an instruction—for instance, turn around, jump three times, and touch your nose. Encourage your child to repeat the instruction and then carry it out.

2. **Find shapes in the landscape around you:** There's a great song that we sing at one of our playgroups—"Oh where oh where has the circle shape gone? Oh where oh where can it be? We are looking for a circle, we are looking for a circle, oh where oh where can it be?" Once you have sung the song, look for a circle. You might find it in a round window, a ball in a shop, etc. When your child has spotted one, sing: "Hooray hooray hooray hooray. We found a circle, we found a circle. Hooray hooray hooray hooray. We found a circle, we found a circle."

3. **Name That Tune:** Hum a song and see if your child can guess what it is.

4. **Hunt the . . . :** Encourage your child to look for something small/big/rough/smooth, etc. If they need help, use the "getting hotter or getting colder" technique. When your child is close, say "hot" and when they're farther away say "cold."

5. **Word association:** Give your child a word like *play* and have them think of an associated word such as *game* or *school*. Carry on taking turns to think of an associated word.

# FIVE ADDITIONAL WAYS TO PROMOTE TALKING . . . ON AN AIRPLANE

1. **Photo Challenge:** Look through the photos on your phone and take turns describing what is happening in each one. Then try to remember what happened before and after each one. I did this with my mum on a recent flight and she was asleep within minutes! Hmmmm . . .

2. **Rhyme Time:** Have some fun rhyming words ("What rhymes with 'dog'?") or making limericks—here's our effort. It's very difficult—try it!

   *There once was a boy from New York*
   *Whose talking skills needed some work*
   *When buying some food*
   *He got in a mood*
   *Because he'd ordered ham and not pork*

3. **No "Nos":** A tricky and fun game for little ones. See what happens when they are not allowed to say yes or no or not allowed to smile. Launch into a barrage of questions usually starting with "Are you ready?" and try and get them to say yes or no, or alternatively say a lot of jokes and try to get them to smile.

4. **Imagine What's Happening Below:** Look out the nearest window and talk about what's happening below: "Do children play on those hills? What's the weather like?" If it's dark, "Are the children sleeping in their homes? I wonder what they look like."

5. **Describe and Guess:** Describe something or someone in the vicinity and have your child guess who or what it is.

## Mastering talking and playing—at the same time!

By about 3 years old, your child will be able to play and talk at the same time—for example, by giving voices to the dolls they're playing with. They'll begin to play in groups with other children, sharing toys and taking turns.

They will also be able to focus on what you say while they're playing, so they won't have to stop what they are doing in order to listen to what you are saying. (The inability to do this is the reason your child sometimes appears to completely ignore you!)

# HOW TO REACT WHEN CHILDREN SAY THE WRONG THING IN PUBLIC

The other day, my friend Jane was walking home with her little one, Grace, and a man walked past them. Grace said very clearly, "Mummy, that was a dirty old man, wasn't it?" He heard and turned around and said something. Jane was mortified and also concerned about where this phrase may have come from. Hopefully, it was just because the man's pants were a bit muddy and Grace obviously had no idea that what she was saying had another meaning.

So, what can you do in these situations? Apart from growing a very thick skin—and a good line in apologies—I would say that it's just a case of accepting it, and at this stage your child has no inhibitions and hasn't yet become in tune with our politically correct culture. For now, all you can do is say, "We mustn't say that, because you might make that man sad." And if you get asked a series of "why" questions about it, answer as best you can, then try to change the subject!

# My child's language has regressed—what can I do?

In some instances, a child's language may pause or sometimes seem to regress, for example, after trauma or change such as the birth of a baby sibling, being immersed into a setting that is not the same language the child speaks, or perhaps you noticed some changes during the pandemic when your child couldn't see other people, like their grandparents.

Here is a short story about Rupa.

Rupa has a 2-year-old daughter and a 5-month-old son. Until her son was born, her daughter was learning new words all the time, but after his arrival it seemed that she went back to baby talk. Rupa came to see me at my drop-in clinic because she was concerned and wanted to know what she could do get her daughter's speech back up to speed.

This is very common when a new baby arrives and the parents' attention is suddenly divided. In toddlers and preschool children (under 5), the resulting "jealousy" may be exhibited by speech regression and attention-grabbing "watch-me" moments during potty-training or play.

As explained, your child might experience a temporary regression of their development in response to the stress, sudden change, or trauma in their family. If you think of development as a set of uneven stairs that children climb as they add on new skills, most children progress in a predictable sequence. But it's possible to take a step backward, find your balance, and then move forward more confidently.

Try not to worry too much. Trust your gut. The best approach is not to become angry or frustrated with your child, but to reward them for using their language skills and give them praise as the older sibling. Time spent around their peers at a playgroup will help model more appropriate language skills, but be careful not to rock the boat again by taking them away from the family. Try to spend some one-on-one time with them every day so that they feel special. It will be difficult to divide your time equally, so don't try, or you will feel added pressure and strain, which your children will pick up on. If you're worrying about a lack of progress, seek professional help.

The very fact that your child is using words functionally to request their needs and wants is a huge telltale sign that bigger and better language development is yet to come and your little one will go from strength to strength. Let's keep the momentum going into chapter 9 and get your little one telling stories like a pro!

Chapter 9

# What to do when . . . your child isn't telling stories

Once your little one is able to say a few sentences, you'll notice how eager they are to build those sentences into little stories. You'll also notice that most of our little ones are born innately sociable and love to chat and interact. Sometimes though, parents might notice that they are not chitter-chattering in longer sentences and trying to expand those sentences into little stories the way some of their peers are. There we go again—the curse of comparison!

We already know that with every new phase of development, new challenges arise. Most children will start talking in longer sentences, use grammar correctly, and begin to master the many irregular patterns of English by the age of 4. Around this time, they'll become much more eloquent when it comes to expressing their feelings and emotions, and they will begin to develop stronger friendships with their peers.

This is also the time when you will begin to think about enrolling your child in elementary school, so in this chapter we'll look at gearing up your child's language skills in preparation for this momentous step. You'll encourage your child to chat more confidently, to listen to and follow complex instructions, and to start to be more eloquent and elaborative with their storytelling.

With this amazing expansion of language comes a child who thinks more deeply and will tell the most compelling stories about their world and how they view it. And, to top this all off, there'll be a sense of humor eruption! So many fun times ahead.

## EXPANDING SENTENCES AND TELLING STORIES

In this stage, your child will already have the basic language skills and you won't have to encourage your child to chat and talk, but remember to stay one step ahead of them—help them to connect their thoughts to words, talk to them about their day, and expand their vocabulary and grammar. Encourage them to talk about everything and anything—to reflect on past and present experiences, plan future events, and predict what might happen, anticipate new experiences, use their imagination to create a fantasy land, and speculate about what they may or may not encounter there.

With so much to talk about, you should expect much longer sentences now, of three or more key words, while your child tries to retell stories of their day or describe their innermost thoughts. Their sentences should be made up of nouns and verbs, sometimes used in the correct tense, and a range of different concepts, all articulated in good sequential order.

In chapter 8 we looked at encouraging your child's emerging narrative skills, and here, we'll learn how to expand them further, in line with the wider range of experiences they are enjoying, the storybooks they are thinking about and the vivid imagination they are developing.

**Top Tip Time** **Expanding sentences and telling stories**

- It's quite hard to retell a story, but even harder to make one up, so start with sequencing a story your child has just read from a familiar book—*The Three Little Pigs* is a good story for this purpose because it's very predictable and has a repetitive phrase in it that makes it easier for a child to hook on to. Read it through together, then allow your child to hunt through the house for objects that tie into the story. Using the props that you collected, go through the book again, talking about each page and each prop. Then take the book away and encourage your child to retell the story once again without any visual support. This will encourage them to retain the new words and attempt to increase their sentence length as they try to retell it.

Next, encourage your child to talk about something that has happened during the day, then something that they experienced in the past, and then something completely made up—this will be progressively harder for them. If they seem to be struggling, help them by expanding their thoughts and words by prompting them to remember key information and modeling the correct versions of their sentences back, fine-tuning the details, adding new words and concepts and correcting grammar.

Continuously encourage your child to tell stories and be increasingly more detailed about the people, places, and times they include in their stories.

- I'm a big fan of show-and-tell, which involves children bringing something in to nursery or preschool to show to the other children and talk about. It can be almost anything—it might be a picture from a newspaper, a feather you found in the park, or a stone from your backyard! If your child has to take something in for show-and-tell, make sure you practice what they'll say at home using the "first, then, and last" technique (see page 183). If there is no show-and-tell planned, why not have a show-and-tell for Daddy or Granny?

- Talk about problems and find different solutions with your child—for instance, "Mummy has lost her keys, so let's think about what we can do . . . phone Daddy, look for them, remember when we last used them, try and pick the lock," or "Oh no, we've run out of milk. Let's think about what to do. . . ."

- Encourage your child to give you a sort of presentation. For instance, you might say, "Tell me all that you know about baseball/Lyn's house/*Sesame Street*."

- Look at textless storybooks such as Raymond Briggs's *The Snowman* and encourage your child to tell the story.

- If you usually read a story while sitting in a particular chair, swap with your child so that they can sit in the storytelling chair.

- Put together some old photographs in a line on the floor and see if, together, you can make up a story.

- Talk about things that happened to you in the past and retell those stories—how lovely it'll be to have a pair of ears to listen to stories from your life. Minnie was always asking Tracey to tell her the story (again!) of when they first got their rescue cat Keith because they had so many mice in their old house.

- Create a storytelling box. Put three or four objects into a box—try an object, a picture of a person, and a picture of a place or an object that represents a place (such as a shovel for the beach), then add any other random object, such as a key, a piece of pasta, a ball, or a clothespin. Try to get your child to make up a story using the contents of the box as inspiration and props. You go first to model the idea for them.

- Buy a photo album and fill it with things you like to talk about—a postcard, pictures of dogs or dinosaurs, the foil wrapper from an Easter egg, a bus ticket, a leaf . . . You could make another one to fill while on vacation or fill one with pictures involving your child's favorite theme (perhaps whales and dolphins, for example).

- Encourage your child to tell stories using puppets (puppets can be quite expensive, so why not take the stuffing out of an old cuddly toy and use it as a puppet?). Teddy could entertain his audience with stories about his visit to the supermarket, the park, or the swimming pool.

## Is my child turning into a liar?
## The make-believe boom

At this stage, children often start telling "lies," especially when they discover that their parents cannot read their minds and that they can cover up the truth (for example, "Did you just eat Mummy's Easter egg?" "No," says little Dexter, with a chocolate-covered mouth).

And it's not just when they've done something wrong and they don't want to admit it. When my niece Eleanor was little, she was always making up stories about what had happened during her day or week. When you asked her a question, she told the truth. It was when she ran out of things to say that she carried on with a pack of lies. My brother was getting increasingly nervous that she was turning into a compulsive liar so he asked for my advice.

My response was that Eleanor was definitely not turning into a liar. She just enjoyed the adult attention and responses to the stories of her day and week and her imaginative brain was running riot, so when she got to the end of the real story, she was so keen to carry on that she made up things rather than end this Special Time.

Children at this age and stage are absorbed in fantasy play and imaginary language and often blur the lines between reality and fantasy when telling a story. The best thing to do is to say, "I really enjoyed it when you told me about what happened at Creation Station—you are so clever to remember that story. And it was funny when you added that extra bit and pretended that the monkey came—it made me laugh." Once you give a child permission to be creative in telling pretend stories, you can always remind them of the distinction between truth and tale, and they can continue with the same amount of engaging enthusiasm.

There'll come a time when your little rascal pretends their tales are real. Sometimes, it's just too irresistible for a 3-year-old not to exaggerate. You can decide how far you let them go with this, but try not to come down and squash their story too early.

If the lying gets out of hand, you might have to clamp down a bit—try not to worry too much, though, because this *is* a normal stage of language development. Let your child's imagination run riot and their language skills blossom. And don't forget to enjoy the fun—I bet you'll struggle not to laugh at some of the tall tales!

## DEVELOPING GRAMMAR

At the same time as listening to a wonderful drama unfold from the mouth of your chatty child (hopefully the kind a movie director will want a piece of one day!) you must also try to notice their grasp of grammar.

The start of grammar development should be well under way. A lot of the basics will have been acquired by now, such as the pronouns (I, you, me, he, she, they); some question words; a basic understanding of the past and future tenses and auxiliaries "he *is* running"; prepositions (in, on, under); and possessives ("the dog's bone"). Gosh, your child has been busy! But there's still a way to go, and by about 4 years, your child will

- learn more prepositions—behind, in front, beside, between (for example, "It's *between* the two books"),
- expand their use of when and why questions (for example, "*Why* are you called 'Daddy'?" and "*When* are you going?"),
- expand their use of the regular past tense (for example, "He played outside"); this begins at 2½ to 3 years,
- learn the irregular past tense (for example, "She *lost* the ball"),
- learn the future tense (for example, "I am *going* to ride a horse" or "She *will* ride a horse") at about 3 to 3½ years, and
- expand their use of possessives—his, hers, theirs—and object pronouns—him, her, them (for example, "That's *his* garden" and "Let's go and see *him*").

We've already discussed a lot of these aspects of grammar, but we haven't yet thought about how we encourage our children to talk about the past or the future. For some ideas, look at the advice in the Top Tip Time that follows.

**Top Tip Time** **Talking about the past**

- After you and your child have done something, immediately ask them to tell you what happened. For instance, as soon as you've washed their face in the bath, say, "What happened?," then model the answer "Mummy washed Jess's face." Just after your child has painted a picture, ask, "What happened?" and wait for the answer—"I painted a picture." If it is not spoken correctly, model it back correctly.

- Find the flash cards you used to illustrate verbs like running, jumping, and eating. Show your child a flash card and say, "What has happened?" instead of "What's happening?" Model the correct past tense—for instance, "The girl jumped" or "Mummy danced"—then encourage your child to take a turn.

- Retell your day or a familiar story using the past tense. Also, act out a story and then retell it again using the past tense.

- Watch what your child is doing—yes, it's the Say What You See technique again! When they have just done something, ask, "What did you kick?," "What do you play with?," or "Where did you wash?" and encourage them to answer in a full sentence: "I kicked the ball," "I played with the doll," or "I washed my face."

**Top Tip Time** **The future tense**

- Again, it's easier for children to learn this tense in the here and now, so use the Say What You See technique. For example, just before you make yourself a drink, as you have a cup held up to the faucet, ask your child, "What is going to happen? Mummy is going to make a drink." Just before your child picks up their favorite toy, say, "Stu is going to play with the LEGO." Then ask what they are going to do next. If they use "gonna," don't worry—we all say this and it makes our language flow more easily.

- Do some cooking and, before you start, talk about all the stages. For instance, you might say, "Let's make some lunch—what about PB&J? What shall we do first? Next? Then? Great, we've got a plan so . . . ready, set . . . cook!"

- Sequencing cards can be a good prop for talking about the future tense. I like the Sequence Rummy Challenge Cards by Trend. Start by using two or three cards, then add more. You can look at the pictures and comment about the sequence of what's taking place in them—for instance, "First she climbs the ladder, then she sits down at the top—what's going to happen next?" Alternatively, make your own sequencing cards by taking photographs, say, of your child going down a slide—the first picture when they're at the top, the next when they've reached the middle, and the last when they're at the bottom of the slide. Then ask them to put the cards in the correct order.

- At bedtime, talk about what will happen tomorrow. For instance, "We've got a big day tomorrow—let's think about what we will do. In the morning, we will buy a birthday present for Tony, then we will come home for some lunch and then we'll go to Tony's party at the swimming pool—yay!"

## QUESTION WORDS—UNDERSTANDING WHY CHILDREN SAY "WHY"

Asking questions is a vital way of obtaining information. Even knowing that a question needs to be asked is quite a step forward for your child—he is acknowledging that he doesn't know something and would like to know about it. Children need to recognize that there is a gap in their knowledge and that they have the ability to ask for help, seek information, or ask for an explanation about something. It's another step in their voyage of discovery—their way of exploring and understanding the world around them.

At this time, children should have learned to use the question words "what," "who," "why," and "where." They will need to practice these words some more—hence the quick recap below—and begin to use new question words such as "when" and "how."

**Top Tip Time** **Question time!**

This Top Tip Time is about encouraging children to ask general questions as well as improving their ability to ask general questions.

- Bring out an object that your child has never seen before and encourage them to talk about it. You could model this by doing a role-play with your partner, with one of you asking the other questions about the object—for instance, "What is that?" and "Where did you find it?"

- Look at holiday photos together and ask questions about them, such as, "Where did we go?," "What did we do next?," "Why were we laughing?," or "Where was Daddy?"

- Give your child a question to ask someone in another room—like a little messenger! For example, you could say, "Ask Daddy where you are going today," or "Ask Nanny what is in the fridge." They will enjoy having the job of asking a question and relaying the response.

### What?

Your child might be able to understand what's meant when asked the question "What's that?"—whether they can answer it will depend on the level of their vocabulary.

Previously, I've advised not asking your child too many questions, but in order for them to start using question words correctly, which is appropriate for this stage of language development, they will have to hear question words being modeled for them. They are older now, so they are likely able to cope with a few questions. Try the following ideas.

- Talk about what you are eating for dinner. You could say, "What are you eating? You're eating [point to your child's food to cue them in] . . . potato, chicken, and peas."

Encourage them to ask you the question back. This may work particularly well on the telephone—if your child is talking to Grandma, who is eating her breakfast or cooking her lunch or dinner, you can whisper to them, "What's Grandma having for dinner?" Hopefully, they will ask Grandma the question and relay the answer back to you. When the phone is hung up you can ask the question again, "What was Grandma having for dinner?" and encourage your child to ask Daddy, "What are we having for dinner?"

- Read books like *The Very Hungry Caterpillar* by Eric Carle or *Handa's Surprise* by Eileen Browne. Both have lots of opportunities for "what" questions—for instance, "What did the caterpillar eat next?"

## Why?

The barrage of whys could commence at any time from about 2½ years, but often enters a whole new league of persistence (and irritation!) when your child is around 3. I imagine every parent of children around this age has had a conversation rather like the following.

Child: "Why are you in the front?"

Adult: "Because I'm driving."

Child: "Why are you driving?"

Adult: "Because we are going to nursery school."

Child: "Why?"

Adult: "Because we can't walk to nursery school; it's too far away."

Child: "Why?"

Adult: "Because it's in the next town over, nearly one mile away."

Child: "Why?"

Adult loses the will to live. . . .

I know it's tempting to turn the tables and ask, "Why do you keep asking me why?" But that will be a bit too advanced for your little one at the moment, so for now you'll have to go with it!

"Why" questions are very often answered with a response beginning "because," so it's important that your child knows how to answer a "why" question appropriately, which you can model for him using these ideas.

- Talk about your day and use the "why/because" format. For example, you could ask, "Why is there a Band-Aid on your knee? Because you scratched it." Then, a few minutes later, act dumb and ask, "Why *did* we put that Band-Aid on your knee? Oh yes . . . [pause], because . . . [pause] you scratched it." If your child doesn't reply in the pause, add the word in for them.

- Make some "why/because" cards—the idea is that they come in pairs to help practice "why" and "because" questions and answers. For example, the first picture might be of a baby crying and the second is of a bottle of milk. You ask, "Why is the baby crying?" and the question, hopefully, prompts the answer shown in the second picture (which starts with "because . . ."): "Because the baby wants milk."

If you don't have time to create cards, just show your child a picture from a magazine or a book and ask a "why" question (for instance, "Why is the girl's dress dirty?" "Because she fell in the mud.").

## Who?

"Who" is one of the easier question words, as it's answered with people's names or animal names, which children generally learn before object names (there are some exceptions to this, though, such as job titles, which are pretty tricky to remember).

- Talk about who is in your family and who is in a friend's family.

- Describe something, (for example, "I have two long ears and a fluffy tail and I love to jump and I eat carrots"), then ask, "Who am I?" Encourage your child to do the same back to you (reverse the roles).

- Talk about characters your child likes from books or TV, then ask questions about them and model answers. For example, you could ask, "Who wears a red dress? Peppa Pig!" or "Who's not in bed? Elmo's not in bed."

- Use the board game Guess Who?, flip up all the characters' frames and ask, "Who has blue eyes, brown hair, and a big nose?" Take turns doing this.

- Read books and ask "who" questions about the characters. For instance, if reading *Who Sank the Boat?* by Pamela Allen, you could keep asking, "Who sank the boat?" or, with *The Gruffalo* by Julia Donaldson and Axel Scheffler, you could ask, "Who lives in the wood?" If you're reading *Dear Zoo* by Rod Campbell, ask, "Who was too grumpy?," and so on.

## Where?

At about age 3, your child should be able to answer "where" questions. This important development will allow them to begin to think about places. When retelling a story, you would naturally have the *when* (the time frame), then the *who* (the person/animal/key character), then the *where* (the place), and then the *what* (what happened). A simple example of this is, "This morning, Auntie May went to the store and bought an apple."

- First, ask your child questions to model the question word "where" in context so they can learn how to ask "where" questions themselves. For instance, you could ask, "Where does a frog live?," "Where does a bird live?," or "Where does Granny live?," then say, "Now you ask me?"

- Play hide-and-seek or hide the thimble and choose such a difficult hiding place that your child has to ask you, "Where are you?" or "Where is it?"

- The *Where's Waldo?* series by Martin Handford is great for practicing taking turns to ask the "where" question.

- Go through a book with your child, simplifying the story by asking questions about it. For example, with the book *We're Going on a Bear Hunt* by Michael Rosen and Helen Oxenbury, you could ask, "Where are the family now?" and encourage them to answer, "In the grass/mud/cave/river."

Then reverse the roles so your child asks you the "where" question and you have to answer. Other books that are good for this activity are *Peace at Last* by Jill Murphy, *Where's Spot?* by Eric Hill and *The Spiffiest Giant in Town* by Julia Donaldson and Axel Scheffler.

## When?

This question word is much more difficult for a child to grasp because, in order to do so, they need to understand the concept of time. That's why being able to answer "when" questions comes much later, at approximately 3½ to 4 years. Use the tips below to encourage this development.

- Ask "when" questions and answer them yourself to create a good language model for your child to copy. For example,

    Q: "When do you need a toothbrush?"

    A: "When you brush your teeth."

    Q: "When do you need a warm coat or a scarf?"

    A: "In the winter."

    Q: "When would you wear these sunglasses?"

    A: "In the sunshine."

- Talk about your day and ask your child questions such as, "When do we have breakfast? Before or after we brush our teeth?"

- Ask your child, "When is your birthday?" and answer for them—for instance, "It's in March."

- Read books like *Owl Babies* by Martin Waddell and Patrick Benson or *The Tiger Who Came to Tea* by Judith Kerr and ask "when" questions (and give the answer, too) whenever a time has been referred to—for instance, "When did Daddy come home? At seven o'clock AM."

# "I FEEL . . .": EMOTIONAL CONCEPTS

It's really important that we teach our children the words they need to express their feelings but, of course, around the 3- or 4-year mark, they are only just learning what a "feeling" actually is. And yet, the emotional highs and lows that children this age experience in any ordinary day are likely to be as unpredictable as sailing the Atlantic Ocean.

Even if they can't yet control or understand their emotions, children at this age definitely have strong feelings about wanting a particular book, not wanting to go to bed, not wanting to get dressed, and not wanting to turn off *Sesame Street*. They get frustrated when they can't reach something that they want to play with or have to wait for something that they want immediately (milk, for instance!). And, if you tell them after the eighth bedtime story that that is the last one, you risk a full-scale meltdown.

Even making choices or decisions can be quite overwhelming for your little one. After years of experience I can still get frustrated about petty things like choosing what to wear in the morning, so imagine how your child may feel about this sort of issue when experiencing it for the first time.

To make matters even more complicated, children cannot control their impulses, so when you say, "Don't do that again!," all they want to do is do it again, either to test your boundaries or to see what the consequences are if they do do it again. I often tell parents to be careful with such phrases. When you say, "Don't run," all your child might hear is "run." Instead, tell them what they *should* do—for example, say "walk!" This is called positive parenting.

There are ways in which you can help your little one to understand their emotions, and learn to express them in a way that won't involve turning bright red and kicking and screaming on the floor. Work through my Top Tip Time games below and you will hopefully have a calmer, more contented kiddo.

## Help your child understand their emotions

Feelings are a bit harder to understand and to learn to say than the other concepts we discussed previously. They are not as tangible as prepositions and, therefore, appear a bit later, toward the 3-year mark. The following games focus on common emotions for young children: happy, sad, angry, scared, and worried. Understanding of feelings such as being bored, excited, surprised, and so on comes later.

Always verbalize and label your child's emotions for them. When they are sad, tell them how they are feeling—for instance, "You are sad because Sarah has gone home, but we'll see her again soon."

Give your child a warning when something they are enjoying is about to end, such as, "In one minute the toys are finished and it's time for bed." But even with advance notice children will usually protest. Explain the feeling your child is having for them by labeling their emotions—for instance, "You are angry because you had to stop playing with Lightning McQueen."

Many children cry and shout when they have to leave a playground, for example. This is normal for a child yet distressing for parents and can often take the shine off a lovely play session. I'd advise mums and dads to put their child's thought into words in such a situation—for example, "You are angry because we had to go home and I am sad because you kicked me." Try to remember that your child was having fun doing things with you, so don't stay away from playgrounds. They are fun and good places to learn skills such as climbing and running—and, in this phase, exploring emotions!

Remember, on this note, to emphasize the positive feelings that the park inspires, too—for instance, "Going down the slide made you laugh!" or "You are so happy on the swing!" When the subject of leaving comes up, you can put a positive spin on that as well by enticing your child with something else interesting—for example, "We are going home to see Daddy and we will be happy when we see Daddy."

If all else fails, get creative with some storytelling that suits your purpose. I have one friend who has invented a tale about a "park man" who comes to lock up the park at the end of each day. If Robert is refusing to leave, my friend simply spots a man in the far distance of the park and says, "Quick, the park man is coming—we'd better leave before he comes or he'll be angry and we'll be sad." Little white lies like this can be the easiest way to diffuse a situation without causing a meltdown.

**Top Tip Time** **Getting a grip on feelings and emotions**

Try the following ideas to encourage your child to grasp emotional concepts.

### Act out feelings

Get your child's favorite dollies or teddies and act out different emotions, such as falling over and feeling sad, then getting angry because they wanted a Band-Aid and then getting bored while Mummy looks for a Band-Aid.

### Make faces

Make faces in the mirror that represent various emotions, saying, for instance, "Let's do a worried face! Now an angry face!" There are some lovely facial expression books available that will help with this—try *Funny Face* by Nicola Smee, which I think is great.

### Seek out examples

When you read books and watch TV with your child, explain and describe how people are feeling. For example, you might say, "Oh dear, Elmo has lost his blanket and he's sad," "Woody is frightened because Buzz thinks he can fly and he might hurt himself," or "Thomas is surprised because the signal has fallen."

# PLAYING WITH LANGUAGE—RHYMING AND JOKING

Now that your child is pretty clever at getting their thoughts and feelings across verbally, it's time to have some real fun! You've giggled at their very cute language mistakes, such as, "Mum, it's soaking hot," or "Peel your eyes open," but now they're really able to make you laugh with some attempts at making up silly jokes, songs, and rhymes. Rhyming and joking demonstrates that your child understands the intricacies of language at a much higher and more abstract level. Here are some ways to encourage your child to play with language.

**Top Tip Time** **Playing with words**

Mess around with words in the following ways.

### Play word-association games

Back in the late 1980s, on a UK children's TV show called *Wacka-day*, there was a clever feature called Mallet's Mallet. The host, Timmy Mallet, would play a word-association game in which you mustn't pause or hesitate when replying, and if you do, you get a bash on the head with a giant foam mallet! Take turns with your child to say words that somehow relate to each other (for example, brick/house/yard or trampoline/jump/hop) until someone can't think of another word to say—at which point you get a bonk on the head.

### Talk about language and how it sounds

Mention onomatopoeia to your child. You needn't use the actual word *onomatopoeia*, but talk to them about words that sound like the object they describe (for instance, "zip," "splash," "roar," and "pop"). Then put them into practice and make the words come alive by zipping a zipper (and stretch out the "zzzzz" sound), making a splash in the water, or popping a bubble. Your child will have to think carefully about this in order to understand the concept.

## Try a story rap

Choose a fairy tale your child knows, find some rhyming words to do with the narrative, and away you go. For example,

> *Jack Jack climbed a beanstalk and back,*
> *to steal a sleeping giant's money.*
> *The giant woke up and didn't think it was funny*
> *and Jack chopped the beanstalk down with an axe.*

## Adding a rhyme

Take turns adding a rhyming word to a line or made-up sentence, such as "the big fat cat sat on the mat and played with a bat" or "the friendly frog sat on a log in a bog and met an ugly hog."

Add on silly rhyming words to basic, everyday objects as a game—your child will probably take great delight in correcting you. So, say, "Can you finish your drinkie-winkie?" and your child will probably say, "No, Mummy, it's not a drinkie-winkie, it's a drink!" Or say, "Can you take off your bib-a-dib-dib?" and you'll be told it's a bib.

## Learning idioms

Teach your child some idioms, which they will probably find highly amusing because the phrases are quite odd when taken literally. See what they think of the following.

> » *Don't cry over spilled milk.*
> » *Many hands make light work.*
> » *Too many cooks spoil the broth.*
> » *Pull your socks up.*
> » *Keep your eyes peeled.*

### Chant rhymes

This rhyme is very popular with most children.

> One two, buckle my shoe,
> Three four, shut the door,
> Five six, pick up sticks,
> Seven eight, lay them straight,
> Nine ten, a big fat hen.

Also try tongue-twisters, and make some up yourself.

## Joking around

One of the best things you can do to develop your child's sense of humor is to use your own. Make jokes, tell funny stories, laugh out loud, laugh at little catastrophes—children love a bit of drama, and tend to respond well to outbursts along the lines of, "Oh dear, I've chipped Daddy's favorite mug," or "Crash, bang, whoops! I've dropped all the baking trays on the floor!"

Having a sense of humor helps children on an emotional and social level, and research shows that people who laugh a lot are healthier because they're less likely to be down in the dumps, which makes them more resistant to illness. And the list goes on—people who laugh more experience less stress, have lower heart rates, pulses, and blood pressure, and have better digestion. Laughter may even help humans better endure pain! So, what can we expect our little ones to laugh at?

Little children tend to have a slapstick sense of humor (they'll love seeing a man with a bucket on his head, a fish wearing sunglasses, or a dog that says "meow") and won't yet be ready to enjoy what we would consider to be a "real" joke.

But what children of this age laugh at the most is toilet humor. Who would have thought bodily functions could be so funny? You have been warned—during this period, an entourage of "pooey," "stinky," "wee-wee," and "fart"-type words will appear. . . .

Gently discourage bathroom humor, or at least try not to participate too enthusiastically (I find that it's the dads who often seem to enjoy it more than the children!). The problem is that once your child works out it's funny, they won't realize that it's not appropriate in certain circumstances—at Great-Aunt Nora's ninetieth birthday party or on the preschool visit, for example. But allow them to laugh a bit—it's harmless and, honestly, my husband, who's in his forties at the time of writing, still thinks a good "poop joke" is hilarious—he assures me it can lighten anyone's mood!

**Top Tip Time** **Playing the joker**

- Encourage your child to find things funny and ensure you laugh heartily at their attempts at humor, too, whether it's drawing "funny" pictures or telling "funny" jokes. Praise them for trying to be funny and be open to surprise—the first time your child makes you laugh is one of life's great pleasures.

- Make humor a part of your day-to-day interactions. Encourage your child to share funny observations or reactions, even when you're around other adults.

- Enjoy funny books, websites, TV programs, and films together. Most children of this age find slapstick humor hilarious; they love watching Daddy Pig from *Peppa Pig* fall into the duck pond or walk into trees. They'll often look to you first to see if they are right that it's funny, so if you giggle, they will inevitably follow suit.

- Teach your child some jokes and encourage them to take center stage and be a comedian. Here are some simple jokes to help.

  » *Why did the banana go to the doctor?*
    *Because he wasn't peeling well!*

  » *What do you call a dinosaur with one eye?*
    *Do-you-think-he-saw-us!*

» *Knock, knock*
  *Who's there?*
  *Lettuce*
  *Lettuce who?*
  *Lettuce in, it's cold out here!*

» *Knock, knock*
  *Who's there?*
  *Boo*
  *Boo, who?*
  *It's okay, you don't have to cry!*

» *What did the policeman say to his tummy?*
  *You're under a vest!*

## CASE STUDY: MINNIE'S FIRST JOKES

When Minnie was little, Tracey invited my husband, Jess, and me over for lunch. Minnie started showing off her counting, trying to get up to ten, and then, out of the blue, created her own joke, saying, "One, two, three . . . chicken!" before collapsing in hysterical giggles. We laughed with her and the more we all laughed, the more encouraged she was to come up with more "jokes"—for instance, "One, two, three . . . cup!," "One, two, three . . . potato!," and "One, two, three . . . dog!" This went on for at least 10 minutes and we were all crying with laughter by the end. It was a real joy to witness a little one begin to experiment with their sense of humor.

# FIVE ADDITIONAL WAYS TO PROMOTE TINY TALKING . . . IN A CAR

1. **I Went on a Picnic and I Brought . . . :** This great memory-building game begins when the first person says, "I'm going on a picnic and I'm bringing . . ." (a food item). Then the second person repeats the first part of the sentence, copies what the first person says, and then adds something of their own. This continues until everyone has had a turn copying what previous people have said and adding their own.

2. **Let's Pretend:** Pretend your car's a different type of vehicle and make up a story about it. "The submarine is being chased by three pink hammerhead sharks." Take turns adding the next sentence or part of the story so that everyone in the car adds something.

3. **Guess Who?:** Describe a person you know or a character from a book or TV show, and have the child guess who you're talking about. Once they do, then it's their turn to describe someone for you to guess who.

4. **Present Time:** When you know it's going to be a long journey, wrap up little presents for your children to open at certain times along the way. Think cheap and simple things like a box of raisins, pipe cleaners to play with, crayons or travel games like Guess Who? The excitement is in guessing what's inside! Ask the children to describe the shape of the parcel, whether it's soft or hard, and what they think might be inside and why.

5. **Car Football:** Everyone in the car chooses an unusual type of vehicle (like a tractor), or a less common color of vehicle (yellow), or a specific type of truck (a gas truck). Whoever sees their chosen vehicle coming toward them scores a point, but if your car overtakes the chosen vehicle, everyone else scores a point. Once someone has seen or overtaken their chosen vehicle, they have to pick a different one. Make up silly words to songs like "The Wheels on the Bus/Truck/Tractor" depending on what type of vehicle you pass.

Now that your little one has mastered the skill of telling stories, there's absolutely no looking back. They're well on their way to becoming the best narrator in town, perhaps heading for a new career in reading!

Remember to keep encouraging your child to work on their ability to sequence their thoughts and to brush up on their grammar. Instead of pointing out a mistake, model back the correct form: "Oh my goodness, you went to the store with Granny? Amazing!"

## Chapter 10

# What to do when . . . your child is shy or reluctant to talk to other people

Most children can become a bit shy or slow to warm up in certain situations no matter how confident they seem to be. This is perfectly natural and often occurs between the ages of 1 and 3 when children become aware of themselves as individuals. Overwhelming shyness might cause a child to close their eyes as an avoidance strategy, cringe if an unfamiliar adult asks them a question, cling to their parent, or look at their parent, praying you'll answer the question for them. Meanwhile you might see other tots in your child's peer group who will willingly chat with anyone and anything—from the snail on the sidewalk or an unfamiliar bus driver, an elderly lady sitting on a park bench, or the boss that even you feel intimidated by. The difference can seem marked but try your hardest not to compare.

In this chapter we'll first try and work out which of the two categories of talking avoidance your child might belong to: reluctant talkers or selective mutism.

# RELUCTANT TALKERS

Being shy, slow to warm up, or intimidated by new people or new situations can stop a child from wanting to talk. We refer to these children as "reluctant talkers" or "reluctant speakers." Do any of these descriptions ring a bell with your child?

- Reluctant talkers present in a similar way at home or in nursery school and will warm up over time, maybe taking only a minute or two.
- Reluctant talkers tend to show their reluctance across all situations they find themselves in, and being quiet and initially withdrawn is part of their personality.
- Reluctant talkers tend to be more cautious about certain personality types, preferring a non-confrontational or sensitive persona as opposed to a director or a disciplinarian type.

## DON'T LABEL YOUR CHILD AS SHY!

Don't refer to your child with a label—for example, "My child is shy"—especially when your child is present. If you do this, your child will be at risk of that label becoming part of their personality. Sometimes parents, as they enter their child's clinic, might say, "Oh, Jay's really shy." When they say that, the therapist will reply, "I'm sure Jay is a fantastic talker!" The goal is to instill confidence in your child and not mark them as shy.

Speech and language therapists are trained to be very good at managing children who are reluctant talkers, the reason being that many children arrive at the clinic feeling a little bit unsure about what is going to happen. Maybe they have been told they're going to see the "talking lady" and the child is consequently thinking, "What demands is this 'talking lady' going to put on me? I'm going to have to talk," and so they feel reluctant. This is especially the case when a little one is already aware that they are struggling with their speech, language or communication skills.

So, when a child enters my room, I never ask them a direct question. I might say, "Wow I love that dinosaur on your shoe. I love dinosaurs, too. I'll show you some of the stegosauruses in my toy box." And because reluctant talkers tend to be happier to chat with less direct, less confrontational, more sympathetic personality types, with a bit of time and patience, they should be chatting happily in a fairly short space of time.

Generally, reluctant talkers will become more confident in finding their voice with the maturity that develops between the ages of 2 and 4. So, as long as they have some friends, and their body language and facial expressions show that they are content with new people given a bit of warming-up time, then I recommend giving them as many opportunities as possible to gain experience in interacting with a range of different people, in many new social situations, and watch and wait for their confidence to grow.

Here are some Top Tip Time strategies to boost your child's confidence to help them to warm up quicker and get them chit-chatting away.

**Top Tip Time** **How can parents help a reluctant talker?**

- Follow your child's lead. You may notice that they are more talkative during certain tasks or activities, especially if they're confident doing them—for example, if they are amazing at puzzles. It sounds obvious, but if they are relaxed and content during these activities, try to provide frequent opportunities for your child to engage in these activities and bring other people into them, too: "Oh, Aunty Lulu, Tai has a new Play-Doh set. You love Play-Doh, too, don't you? Would you like to see it?"

- During your daily Special Time, provide extra time for your child to produce a response. If it is whispered, that's fine to start with. If you didn't hear what they said, indicate that you are having some trouble hearing and suggest that the problem is yours: "I didn't quite hear that. I must need to clean my ears out!" Don't ask for a repetition yet.

- Give them the opportunity to fill in the rest of your sentence by filling in the blank. For example, "Then the little pig said, 'Not by the hair of my . . .'" If your child only makes an animal noise or sound effect, recognize that this is an attempt to communicate and praise the child for a correct or appropriate response. "That was a great pig noise. I can do one, too. Oink-oink."

- Act as though they did speak, and respond to the unspoken remark. For example, if you give them something, you say, "Thank you," then say, "You're welcome." This is not meant to be sarcastic—you're just modeling appropriate conversation to encourage talking!

- Encourage guessing. It takes the right/wrong edge off the response. "Guess what we're having for dinner?"

- Create situations where your child is likely to talk. For example, hold the book upside down to read it, or "forget" to give them something they need, like a spoon for their yogurt. The words will hopefully just pop out! (See communication temptations, page 289.)

- Use Say What You See (pages 24–26). Model language while your child is busy with an activity. Talk about what they are doing and the items they are using. "You've got the biggest, fattest marker and you're doing circles on the paper." You're not expecting a response here—and that's important because it takes all pressure off—but your child will hear the words and sentences that match the activity they're doing.

- Reward speech efforts immediately at the right level for the child (some children don't like over-the-top praise). Praise from a parent is a very powerful reward! "Good job. You've got a beautiful voice."

## Avoid the following . . .

- Do not insist that your child speak, and don't punish them for not speaking.

- Do not withhold toys or food until they speak. This could start them on a pattern of becoming withdrawn or angry, and it could escalate to a battle for control between them and you or other authority figures, such as teachers.

- Don't talk about your child's speech in front of them. Avoid saying things like "They don't talk." "You must talk today; it would make Mummy so happy." This will only put added pressure on them to speak.

## When is it a problem or time to get special help?

- When your child is not communicating with others in their own home or is unable to talk in situations outside the home, it is time to get help. It is important to know that this is not a case of "will not talk" but of "cannot talk" due to fear and anxiety.

- If the periods of silence at nursery school have gone on longer than six to eight weeks, get some help.

- Anxiety becomes a problem when it interferes with everyday life, which is the case with selective mutism (see the following), and therefore it needs to be addressed. Many parents say that from an early age they could tell their child was anxious and they had hoped their child would grow out of it. Others might have thought the anxiety their child showed was normal; perhaps they were similar as children.

- Inquire about the preschool speech and language services in your area. If your child has started nursery school, contact the classroom teacher and ask about an assessment for speech and language services and to set up a meeting so everyone is on the same page.

## SELECTIVE MUTISM

Now that we've learned about reluctant talkers, let's turn to another cohort of children, those who are so anxious about new social situations and new people that their bodies almost freeze in panic, and they physically cannot speak. This is called selective mutism.

Selective mutism is fundamentally an anxiety disorder—a phobia of speaking in certain situations. Generally children with selective mutism have a lot to say and are keen to say it, but just can't. They can talk quite happily and freely in some situations, such as when they're at home with their parents, but completely freeze—both verbally and sometimes physically—in others.

I suspect you have had that feeling yourself of being overcome with emotion or nerves, and your throat tenses up and you get that strangled feeling that keeps you from being able to speak or swallow. This happened to me recently, at my auntie's funeral, where I had to give a speech, and every time I opened my mouth to speak, I couldn't. I was overcome with emotion. Imagine having this horrible feeling pretty much the whole time you're at nursery school! It's debilitating and tiring, and once that panic reaction is set in motion, it's hard to stop and becomes habitual.

There are two types of selective mutism: high-profile selective mutism and low-profile selective mutism.

## High-profile selective mutism

In high-profile selective mutism, children won't communicate or participate in a particular environment at all. They stay silent and passive (or sometimes even frozen) throughout.

Picture a child who does not say a word at school and remains passive even to the extent that an adult might have to put their coat on for them at playtime. But the exact same child is perfectly willing to be independent and chat freely when at home. The child's anxiety is tangible, and relatively easy to detect, because the child simply *can't* speak.

## Low-profile selective mutism

Children with low-profile selective mutism might be able to answer direct questions by whispering or speaking softly, perhaps with their head lowered—for example, they might answer the teacher in a very quiet voice. This is predominantly because they are rule abiders; they like to be compliant and therefore have a very strong desire to please the adults they are communicating with.

A child with low-profile selective mutism would never speak spontaneously by initiating a conversation, requesting something, or sharing information in the environment where they feel the anxiety. This might be in a particular social situation, usually nursery school, or with a particular person. Conversely, they will chat happily with peers or parents at home, perhaps on the playground or when the children have gone off to wash their hands for snack time. Low-profile selective mutism is far harder to identify because the child can and is speaking, but only on their own terms.

In both kinds of selective mutism, a child might present with some other characteristics, such as the following.

- Blank facial expressions
- Not being able to look at the people they are communicating with
- Frozen appearance in body posture; body tension
- Excessive tendency to worry
- Difficulty initiating play with other children
- Being anxious. Sometimes when we take a developmental history from parents of children who have selective mutism, we find that anxiety runs in the family.

Triggers of selective mutism can include the transfer from home to nursery or from one room or class to another within the same setting. Sometimes a loss or trauma can trigger selective mutism. (Seek help from a psychologist if you think this is the root cause of the selective mutism).

Children with selective mutism are different from children who are language delayed or those who have a social communication disorder, such as autism (see page 274). Children who are language delayed can't talk, though they want to and need help learning how. Children who have a social communication disorder can talk but don't understand the need to talk in a social situation.

And children with selective mutism are children who can talk but won't talk. In some cases they are desperate to talk and don't want to be quiet, but they clam up every time they are required to speak. Please note: It is also possible to have a dual diagnosis of selective mutism and autism or language delay and selective mutism.

From the periphery, it can be difficult for family members or close friends. The child's inability to speak can make them frustrated or confused as to why the child won't speak to them. It can even feel like a personal attack—*little Johnny is choosing not to speak to me. Why doesn't he like me?* But let me remind you, this is not a choice, it is a whole-body fear, an automatic response to a stressful situation that the child has no control over, and this is what stops them from talking.

---

## SELECTIVE MUTISM FACTS

- In 2015, researchers Maggie Johnson and Alison Wintgens described selective mutism as "a phobia of talking or being expected to speak or being heard to speak by others."

- A child with selective mutism has to be talking and communicating effectively in one environment but not in another, and this pattern has to go on for at least one month. The most common scenario seen in children is those who are chatting happily at home but are silent or nearly silent at nursery school.

- The onset of selective mutism is typically between 2 and 4 years of age.

- More girls are affected than boys.

- It is a relatively rare disorder affecting about 1 in 140 children. These odds mean that many of you with concerns in this area can be reassured that your child is a reluctant talker rather than selectively mute (the latter is far more serious).

- Selective mutism is more common in certain groups of children—with language delay, speech delay/disorder, and bilingualism, for instance.

- Selective mutism is related to high levels of anxiety and sometimes anxiety runs in families.

**Top Tip Time** **How can we help children with selective mutism?**

First, look out for signs that your child is anxious. These might be

- changes to or difficulty with sleeping or eating,
- changes in behavior, such as more tantrums, becoming more physical, etc.,
- increase in avoidance, as in avoiding activities the child might have previously enjoyed,
- physical symptoms such as stomachache, feeling sick, headache, etc.,
- seeking more reassurance than you would usually expect, and/or
- seeming withdrawn or quieter than usual.

How can we lower anxiety and increase self-esteem? Here are some general tips for children who struggle with anxiety.

- Help your child communicate how they feel. Every time your child feels an emotion, label it for them. Teach your child that you can feel an emotion in your brain and in your body; teach them its name and how the emotion makes your body feel.
- Validate your child's feelings. Whatever emotion your child feels, let them know that it's okay to feel that emotion and that you're there for them and that they're doing a really good job.
- Help them feel safe. Perhaps you could also set up a safe space for them at home or school (for example, a den or quiet room they can access to seek comfort when they are feeling anxious).
- Help them feel like they have some control. Your child might be feeling like things are out of their control. You could help your child focus on things they *can* control (for example, what food they have for lunch).
- Help them regulate their emotions. Encourage your child to do more calming or sensory activities, like coloring or Special Time, when they seem anxious/overwhelmed (for example, when they get home from school).

- Recognize anxiety in yourself. If you, the parent, suffer from anxiety, try to get help by seeing a psychologist.

- Think about problem and reaction sizes—some children can react disproportionately to a problem. Talk about this. An extreme example of a younger child whose cookie just broke (tiny problem for the parent and major problem for the child) versus a child who ran across the road without looking (major problem for the parent and a tiny problem for the child). Try to map out the day, locating where problems might occur and talk about strategies that might help.

- Be predictable and try to make your day predictable, too, by using a visual timetable and talking about what's going to happen. Prepare for any changes.

- If your child has separation anxiety when you drop them at nursery school, which is fairly typical for children between 6 months and 3 years old, always say goodbye and always make goodbyes positive: Smile and wave, hug and kiss, tell them you'll be back and that you love them dearly, even if they cry. Don't think the best thing to do is drop them off, distract them, and make a run for the exit. No! This will only make the separation anxiety worse and could even trigger separation anxiety 24-7, because they'll be desperate to cling on constantly out of fear that when you put them down, there's a chance you'll suddenly disappear.

- If a particularly unusual or shocking event has occurred, talk about it.

- Try figure-8 breathing. Draw a sideways number 8 on a piece of paper. Put your child's finger on the place where the two circles meet. As they breathe in, trace their finger over one circle, and as they breathe out, trace their finger over the second circle. Keep going until they feel calmer.

- Use the distraction technique; for instance, when my daughter felt reluctant to go to school when we lived in France, after we'd talked about it and I'd acknowledged her feeling, I crazily gave her a piece of chewing gum—even worse, it was Hubba Bubba. My mum would have gone mad but it does work! Allowing her to chew on something felt comforting and broke the habitual "school run" anxiety, making it so much easier!

## What to do ... if your child isn't talking at school

Don't delay—arrange an appointment at school and go through this list with your child's teacher. That would be a great first step.

The teacher should do the following.

- Acknowledge your child's condition and make a nonverbal connection with them by playing a range of nonverbal games. You could try pairs or Connect 4. This is critically important for the long-term prognosis.
- Create a communication-friendly environment in the classroom and accept all attempts to communicate, including whispers, gestures, and eye contact.
- Prepare and practice what the child will do ahead of a social situation at school: For taking attendance, arrange for the child to hold up a card that says, "Good morning," and for telling news about the weekend's activities, ask the parents to bring in pictures of what the child did, and so on.
- Build confidence through predictable daily routines.
- Appoint a member of staff to help—someone who is sympathetic, who understands selective mutism, and who doesn't think the child is playing a game or being manipulative or misbehaving by not speaking. I promise I have heard staff say these sorts of things.
- Increase opportunities to access safe and secure social situations to communicate in—for example, set up a little tent in the calm space in the classroom, or have a few quieter children play together on the climbing frame in the garden.
- Use loud instruments in music that would drown out the sound of the child's voice, making it easier for them to try to make a sound. Encourage communication through the instruments.

- Push for participation in noisy group activities such as singing, chanting, or vocalizing as animals.
- Encourage the use of bigger, stronger actions or roles in mime, movement, or dance.
- Use puppets in play or drama.
- Give the child jobs and responsibilities. Encourage the child to run errands with another child at first.
- Ask you to bring in a a video or recording of your child talking at home so that the teachers and peers can see and hear them talking.
- Encourage lots of playdates.
- Instead of relying on words, try showing showing a picture, writing on a whiteboard, or acting out a response, allowing your child to select from a set of alternative responses (these could be verbal responses, written words, objects, or pictures) or allowing them to work in a pair listening and responding together.
- Do things with, rather than for, the child, ensuring that the child is the one to complete the task.
- Build relationships with the child themself and their peers and other adults—for example, by keeping the other children included in any small group activities you have with the child.
- Use a gesture to accompany responses for all children in the class. The child then has a means of contributing to activities other than using spoken language. Encouraging all children to use the gesture while giving a verbal response ensures the child is not singled out.

# CASE STUDY: MY CHILD WON'T TALK AT NURSERY SCHOOL

"My three-and-a-half-year-old daughter, Elina, has been attending nursery school five mornings a week for three months and has not uttered a word to anyone while she is there (even the teaching staff). She went to playgroup (one where I left her) two mornings a week the year before. No speech there, either, although I didn't know this until recently—they just thought she was shy. I had no idea about any of this as she speaks normally when she's at home or anywhere other than nursery school! As she starts full-time school in a few months, this is now becoming worrying. What can I do?"

This sounds like a fairly classic case of selective mutism. It can be pretty tricky to overcome, unfortunately, so it is important to try to crack it early in Elina's school career, so her parents need to get the right people involved as soon as possible. Here is my advice on how to handle this issue.

- First, take all pressure off the child to talk and tell the nursery staff to do so, too. Saying things like "You can't have a drink until you say 'drink'" or "I'll be angry if you don't talk" won't improve the situation.

- Start by placing a person she will talk to (maybe the key staff member—parents are often too emotionally involved with the situation and this can sometimes be noticed by the child) in the setting with her, every day if possible, even if it is just for a short period of time. If it can't be the key staffer, try another sensitive member of staff that Elina seems to respond to.

- Ask the adult to take the child to a quiet area somewhere in the nursery or, ideally, in a separate room attached to the nursery. Let them play together using a nonverbal game (for example, Hungry Hungry Hippos or a puzzle), for about 10 minutes every day. Don't ask any questions or give any reaction if she speaks. If she whispers, don't encourage her to say it more loudly. Do this every day until she has started to talk.

- Then allow either another member of staff or another child to join in and play games. All play the game together. Once spoken communication is established in the side room with a number of children, encourage Elina to play the same games back in the main nursery, then build up to a group dynamic again.

- If a side room isn't available, allow Elina to whisper to the key staff members and then slowly extend the distance away from the talk partner so that Elina can be overheard by others, although she isn't talking to them. Gradually, expand the number of talk partners and others allowed to overhear until she is able to speak freely.

- Sometimes, an inanimate talk partner (such as a teddy or other soft toy) can be used at first, so that in the setting Elina is talking into a soft toy's ear—although the teddy doesn't respond! This would need to be on Elina's agenda and she would probably need to want to speak, or she wouldn't be motivated to break this situation.

- To help motivate her, talk to her about how lovely it will be when she is able to speak at school, without pressuring her. Just put the idea into her head that one day she will be able to speak in school and how great that will be. Don't ever talk about how she doesn't talk while she's in earshot.

- If these strategies don't help, consulting an educational psychologist would be a good next step.

## Selective mutism and bilingualism

If your child is bilingual and going into a setting where the language is completely different from their own, it's normal to go through a silent period. For some children, this can be quite short but, for many others, it can last a few months as their ear becomes attuned to the new language they're immersed in, and they become more confident to try to speak it.

I have first-hand experience of this. We moved to France for a year when Jess was 5 years old. She was confident and bright in her English school, and we slotted her into the local French school without a second thought.

In the first few weeks, we knew she wasn't finding the language easy, which was perfectly reasonable. But after a month, my husband was asked by her teacher, "Does your daughter speak?" Fairly mortified, especially that I hadn't been more on top of it, we began to work with the teacher to implement a few strategies.

- Praise all attempts to communicate, including gestures, signs, whispers, etc.
- Simplify your language when you speak to a bilingual child, and perhaps learn some key words and phrases in their own language, backing them up with gestures where possible.
- Give choices using visuals so they can immediately copy the language you use.
- Use closed questions that require a yes or no answer.
- Don't correct any of their attempts, even if you know they're not quite right.

Implementing these strategies took the pressure off Jess to talk, and after another couple of weeks, she began to talk in single words and short phrases, using the most beautiful French accent. Phew!

For more on bilingualism, see page 253.

The time to be concerned is when the silence is more sustained and more consistent and persistent in certain environments. The general rule is that if the silent period goes on longer than four months, seek help from an SLP.

As I've mentioned, even for adults, going through periods of stress or anxiety might give us a lump in our throat, perhaps a dry mouth or an increased heart rate, making our breathing faster and deeper. All of which make it harder—or nearly impossible—to get our words out. These are the physical responses brought about by our internal feelings and emotions and this "Fight, Flight, Freeze" is a very real and debilitating reaction to anxiety. And we have absolutely no control over it—they are automatic and subconscious responses to external stimuli.

Before the COVID-19 pandemic, the number of children diagnosed with anxiety or anxiety-related disorders was rising, but post-pandemic this has skyrocketed. So, when we take all of this into consideration, perhaps we can start to understand why anxiety-related language problems like selective mutism are becoming increasingly common in children. The number of children with anxiety/selective mutism seems to be shooting up, and the earlier we can step in to help the better. In this scenario, watch and wait is not an option!

# Chapter 11

# Other Common Concerns

# WHAT TO DO IF YOUR BABY HAS TONGUE-TIE

Everybody seems to be talking about tongue-tie at the moment—it's often blamed for feeding problems at birth (as some people believe it could prevent the baby from latching on properly) and speech delay in children. So, what is it?

Look in the mirror and stick your tongue up toward the roof of your mouth. You will notice a flap of skin that joins the underside of your tongue to the floor of your mouth. In cases of "true" tongue-tie, this flap of skin (called a frenulum) extends right to the tongue tip, which restricts the tongue so that it cannot protrude beyond the front teeth or reach back to the far molars to clean them after a meal. In extreme cases, this "pulling" at the tongue tip forms a heart or bulb shape.

While true tongue-tie affects a small percentage of newborns (recent reports suggest about 5 percent[1]), a large majority will have an element associated with tongue-tie. And this is where the problem lies. Some people immediately blame the tongue-tie for latching difficulties, whereas a poor latch can be caused by a whole range of factors, including reduced muscle strength or coordination in the mouth, positioning, and difficulty turning the head to one side, to name a few. Concerned parents may also believe or be led to believe that tongue-tie can hamper or delay speech. And both of these reasons are used to explain why the baby needs "the snip."[2]

A minor operation in which a pair of blunt-ended sterilized scissors are used to snip into the frenulum to free the tongue may be suggested. Once the frenulum is snipped, the baby is put to the breast instantly so that the milk can work its antibacterial and anti-inflammatory magic and the adviser can see the baby's new feeding action and help Mum to position correctly for the "perfect" latch.

I didn't realize that tongue-tie diagnoses were so rife until I had problems with feeding myself (and, let's be frank, who doesn't?). When Jess was about a week old and breastfeeding was a painful nightmare, I was told that Jess had a tongue-tie, creating a click when she was feeding, which led to air entering her mouth, causing a latching problem. I was amazed. I could see instantly that Jess was not tongue-tied. In fairness, she did have a very slight bulb shape at the end of her tongue, but it clearly wasn't restricting her movement, as she could move her tongue into a flat shape and even beyond her lips at times. In fact, it turned out that poor Jess had oral thrush, and because of the furry coat it gave her tongue, she could not feel when the nipple was inside her mouth and couldn't get a good latch, especially as her mouth was feeling uncomfortable and possibly painful.

Luckily, I was confident in my convictions—but only because it's my profession. If I hadn't been an SLP, with the continuous worry a new mother feels, I would have probably ended up getting Jess's tongue snipped and putting her through an unnecessary and sometimes costly operation.

In another case, a friend of mine who's a nurse was also told her baby was tongue-tied, causing feeding problems. She was so desperate to get feeding back on track that she scheduled the operation immediately, and to this day she is convinced that this procedure, to snip the tongue free, did make all the difference. I am not so sure—I think it was probably the two hours of breastfeeding coaching after the operation that did the trick.

Lots of professionals are advocating the snip zealously, as if it were always necessary and as if tongue-tie were the obvious cause of speech and/or feeding problems. One study looked at 115 babies who on average were 1 month old.[3] All had been referred for the surgical procedure but 63 percent were able to successfully breastfeed with the help of specialists, including speech and language pathologists. The number of cases being referred for this procedure has increased dramatically with seemingly little data to back it up.

So, what about speech? Even if the tongue is tied all the way to the tip, research supports that this does not have any bearing on articulating speech sounds. Despite the tongue-tie, the tongue can still move around the mouth into all of the positions necessary to articulate all of the sounds in the English language. Therefore, tongue-tie is not a cause of speech-sound difficulties, so the snip is not a solution for speech-sound problems.

With regard to feeding problems, I would be overstepping my field of expertise (and, therefore, as guilty as the professionals who advocate the snip as a solution for alleged speech-sound difficulties) if I were to take a bold stance. However, my view is that most babies have feeding difficulties in the first two or three weeks, with many different causes. To believe that the snip is a panacea for every kind of problem is very simplistic. Amazingly, at least half of my prenatal group of eight were told to get their babies' tongues snipped even though, when I examined them, there was absolutely no sign of a tie at all.

So, even if you are desperate for an answer to feeding difficulties in those early few weeks, I'd advise you to think carefully about a tongue-tie snip. There may not be any lasting damage as a result of having this minor operation (although the snip could cut through a blood vessel, leading to bleeding and pain, and the tongue may feel loose for the baby afterward, which can cause the little one to gag and cough), but why pay a great deal of money for a procedure that isn't always necessary? I believe that a lot more research needs to be carried out regarding this matter because the current default advice to get the snip is unconvincing and worrying.

# WHAT TO DO IF YOUR CHILD WON'T GIVE UP THEIR DUMMY

Dummy or not? There is no universal rule, but everyone seems to have a very strong opinion about it. So, what do the professionals say?

You may be surprised to hear that there are some situations in which an SLP would recommend a dummy to strengthen the mouth and help a child establish a good suck for feeding in the very early stages. At other times, a child with significant speech-sound difficulties might visit an SLP for an assessment. An experienced practitioner would know immediately that the child sucks a dummy, on account of the shape of their lips, teeth, and tongue or the child's excessive drooling. It would not be unusual for the SLP to refuse to see that child again until they no longer use a dummy. Sucking on a dummy can restrict the movements of the lips and tongue, causing major difficulty in articulating sounds.

We all know that babies like to suck, and dummies can help them to self-soothe at nap times or when they are tired or grumpy. But regular or constant use of a dummy can hamper your child's speech, simply because a child is likely to start talking with a dummy in their mouth, restricting the movement of their tongue, lips, and jaw and encouraging bad habits to develop even when the dummy is not in their mouth. (This is different from thumb-sucking, as a child who sucks their thumb will usually take their thumb out of their mouth to speak.) Take the "t" sound, for instance. It is articulated by moving your tongue upward in the mouth to touch the ridge behind your top teeth. This sound is pretty impossible to make when a massive obstacle is in the way, so the child might say "k" instead and, therefore, "toe" becomes "koe."

The general rule is that once a child starts attempting words, you should start to think about ditching the dummy. So, if your child reaches roughly 18 months and is showing signs of being hooked on their dummy, my advice would be to take the dummy away completely rather than trying to reduce the number of hours the dummy is used, which is what some parents try at first.

At my clinic we find that parents have a good success rate when they tell children to leave their dummy out on their birthday or at Christmas for Santa, who will leave them a present in return. Another trick is to visit a young baby and persuade your child to give the dummy to the little one, saying, "You are so kind, the baby needs it much more than you." Every time your child asks for it after that, you say again, "How kind you are, you gave it to baby . . ."

Dentists agree that dummies have a significant impact on the development of children's teeth. When choosing a dummy, a dentist would suggest, aside from not having one at all, that you go for an orthodontic design, with a hole in the teat, which is supposedly better for the teeth. But with speech, they are all equally restrictive to the movements of the mouth, so neither one is better.

Through my work, I have met lots of families who use the dummy as a noise dampener. If your baby is being noisy, under no circumstances should you be tempted to use a dummy as a gag. If your baby is intolerably vocal, this might be annoying when you can't hear a conversation or the TV over the din, but it is good news that they are making lovely noises and it's best to encourage their "speech," not restrict it. Babies from large families or generally noisy environments will babble loudly to compete. So, if you have a noisy baby, check whether the environment is too loud for them before muffling the sound with a dummy.

## CASE STUDY: FOUR-YEAR-OLD DUMMY USER WITH SPEECH PROBLEMS

When a child comes into the clinic I can see immediately by the shape of the mouth if the child uses a dummy. I recall one 4-year-old boy who kept the front of his mouth completely still while talking—even his teeth were stunted in growth due to dummy interference. Parents tend to put the dummy away as they walk into the health center but I knew instantly what the problem was. To be technical, he was using the back of his mouth to talk, getting into a habit of saying "k" and "g" instead of "t" and "d" ("t" and "d" are tongue-tip sounds, while "k" and "g" are made using the back part of the tongue) and he had a *dental lisp*, meaning that his tongue appeared between his front teeth to say the "s" sound. He would say "key" instead of "tea," and he would use the Welsh "ll" sound (as in "llanelli") instead of "s," so "sausages" would be spoken as "llaullagell." He was beginning to be aware that he didn't sound like his friends and was getting frustrated. It was no surprise to the mother when I told her to ditch the dummy immediately, and within a couple of months, his speech was almost perfect. His mum explained that letting go of the dummy involved a couple of nights of crying but had been a lot easier than she ever expected.

## WHAT TO DO IF YOU FIND YOURSELF SAYING "NO" ALL THE TIME

You really don't want your child's first word to be "no," although I must stress that this is very common and it doesn't mean that all their experiences so far have been negative; it's just such an easy word for a tiny tot to say, and despite your best intentions, you may have said "no" quite a lot!

But wouldn't you rather your child's first utterance was "bike" or "Mummy"? If so, when your little one starts throwing food on the floor, pulling their friend's hair, biting your finger, chasing the dog, crawling away when you're trying to change their nappy, or rearranging their grandmother's favorite fine bone china, you have to think hard about how to manage the situation. At about 10 months, a baby's memory starts to improve dramatically, and they begin to retain the new words you say to them. So, instead of saying, "No," you have to think of something different to say. My advice follows.

Choose your battles. In other words, if your baby wants another cookie when you're visiting relatives and you want to avoid a meltdown, then hand it over! It's just not worth battling over every issue—and getting stressed and upset yourself. If you are going to refuse, you must stick to your guns or your little one will quickly realize that their tears and tantrums get them their own way and, next time, will immediately launch into the tantrum, knowing that it worked last time.

Remember that when you scream, "No! No!" in a high-pitched, loud, and energetic way it can be mistaken for a great game and actually reward the very thing you've said "no" to, encouraging your baby to do it again to get the same fun response.

So, decide what you DO want to be strict about—whether it's not throwing food on the floor at mealtimes (so that you can confidently take your baby out for lunch, knowing they won't leave a trail of devastation behind them!), not pulling hair (be it other babies' or pets'), or not pulling Granddad's glasses off his face.

Also, I encourage mums and dads to try "positive parenting" and tell their children what they *want* them to do, not what they don't want them to do. Here are some examples.

- "Quiet voice now, please," instead of "No screaming!"
- "Not for Ben" or simply "Stop!," rather than "No, Ben" when he tries to put a stone in his mouth, as you quickly replace the stone with a ball or a rattle (also known as the distraction technique).
- Say, "Gently," instead of "No!" when your little one tugs at the dog's tail or pulls out your dad's last remaining lock of hair.
- If getting dressed always causes tantrums, turn it into a game by saying, "I'm going to catch your hand!," "I'm going to catch your leg!," or "Hello, hand" (as it emerges from a sleeve), or "Hello, foot" (as it pops out of a pants leg) instead of simply saying, "No, Aida, will you lie still!"

If your child keeps doing things that require you to think or say "No!," you might need to ask yourself why. "Naughty" is a surface term to describe behaviors we can see on the outside that are the result of something that's happening on the inside. To put this a different way, all behavior is communication. What are the reasons why this behavior is happening? You have to dig deep, observe, and discuss with other key people—your partner, the grandparents, or other parents with children of a similar age. Sometimes poor behavior is a cry for attention. You know what to do . . . a daily Special Time will work wonders, I promise!

## WHAT TO DO IF YOUR BABY WON'T GIVE UP THE BOTTLE

Health professionals recommend that a baby should begin to give up the bottle at 12 months. This is the start of a process that parents manage in different ways. Some stop using the bottle immediately and give a sippy cup or an open cup right away, while others reduce over time the number of bottle feedings a child has over the course of a day. Prolonged use of the bottle or dummy causes irreparable damage to the shape of the mouth (which affects speech development), in the following ways.

- Just behind your top teeth, there is a hard surface called the alveolar ridge, which is very important for clear and precise speech, in particular the "t," "d," "s," "n," and "l" sounds. If you suck on a bottle over time, the shape of the ridge is affected and there is less room for the tongue to articulate against it to form clear speech sounds.

- When you suck from a bottle your lips and tongue curl around the teat, forming a round shape to the lips, which can become habitual even when the bottle is no longer in the mouth. This shape is detrimental to good clear speech—for instance, try saying "f" when your mouth is curled into this shape.

- When you suck on a bottle or dummy, the middle section of your tongue becomes strong and, therefore, more dominant when articulating speech sounds. However, it is the tongue tip that needs to be the most agile when it comes to articulating sounds. When the middle part of the tongue takes over, the tongue tip pokes through the front teeth, forming a lisp. The words sound slushy and imprecise as in the case of Chris Eubank or Jamie Oliver, who have a dental lisp.

When I tell parents at my clinic about the harmful effect prolonged use of the bottle may have on their child, they commonly say, "Well, they only have it once every day before bed." My response is, "If I were to do a set of sit-ups every day, I'd have a wonderfully flat stomach." Even one daily repetition can make a big difference to muscle and structural development of the mouth. So, . . . banish the bottle now!

**Top Tip Time** **From bottle to sippy cup**

I advise parents to move to an open cup as soon as possible after the age of 12 months, or earlier, if you have the inclination. A receptacle that pours is always best. (Avoid those that demand a suck—this swirls the fluid around the teeth. Also, the mouth position for sucking is not one to encourage—try sucking as you read this and you will notice that the bottom sections of your cheeks get pulled in, causing your lower jaw to become misaligned with your top teeth, making it very hard to speak clearly. This is known as an overbite.)

- **If you're giving an open cup (one without a lid), help your child to tilt the cup up for drinking and down for pauses, and try to maintain contact between the rim of the cup and your child's bottom lip at all times.** Using a constant, predictable rhythm will also help. Another tip for when you first move to an open cup is to use thicker fluids that are less runny, such as a fruit smoothie, so it's easier for your baby to keep them in the cup. Developmentally, a child should be able to hold an open cup from 12 months with only a little spillage.

If going straight to an open cup fills you with fear (I totally understand that no one likes the idea of milk being spilled all over their carpet or pajamas), take the natural first step and try a sippy cup, which is much better than a bottle.

- **When choosing a sippy cup, the spout should be short to ensure that the fluid is tipped just inside the lips, which will, in turn, encourage the tongue to dip down to the base of the mouth to make a cavity to receive the fluid.** This is a better position for tongue movement and, therefore, speech development. Watch to see if your toddler's tongue is sticking out under the sippy cup spout. If so, find a fatter, shorter-spouted sippy cup.

  Straws are always great for creating a good tongue position in the mouth. You can buy sippy cups that have straws already attached, but the straws tend to be quite long, which makes it harder for little ones to actually suck up the fluid. Otherwise, try a carton with a straw or simply a cup with a straw.

Avoid non-spill valves, which encourage tongue thrust. These types of sippy cup are almost as bad as a bottle.

---

### CASE STUDY: A BOY ADDICTED TO HIS BOTTLE

Recently, I worked with an 18-month-old boy named Saif who drank only from a bottle—not just his bedtime milk, but all his drinks during the day, too. He had a significant lisp. Not only was the "s" sound spoken with his tongue between his teeth, but many other sounds were, too—the "t," "d," "n," "sh," "j," and "ch" were all spoken with his tongue sticking out. I gave his instructor at nursery school, Jude, some tips. (It was decided the activities should be carried out at school, as Saif was there full time, and his mum had three other children, making it difficult for her to find time for practice at home). Jude worked really hard to wean Saif straight on to an open cup. Here are the techniques she used.

- Helping him learn to hold the open cup
- Encouraging him to watch the other children drinking

---

- Giving lots of praise when he held the cup to his lips

- Playing with open cups in the home corner of the nursery, and helping the teddies to drink from them

- Telling the Mr. Tongue story (page 273)

- Doing the Bigmouth tongue exercise program, which consists of a set of pictures showing a tongue pointing up and down, moving from side to side, and poking in and out. These were conducted when Saif looked in the mirror in the children's bathroom every time he washed his hands. Also, Saif's mother was given the same pictures.

- Sticking pictures of the tricky sounds around the mirror (for example, a snake for "s") and encouraging him to say these sounds with his teeth metaphorically stuck together so his tongue didn't pop forward

There was a big improvement in Saif's speech, but then the summer vacation arrived. Saif's mum hadn't yet managed the switch from bottle to sippy cup at home (even though he'd managed this at nursery school) and gave him a bottle whenever he made a fuss.

When Saif returned to nursery school in September, his lisp was back with a vengeance. It really stood out to Jude and me, and we honestly couldn't believe how much worse his speech was. It completely reinforced the message of the importance of bottle versus cup-drinking and how we needed better persuasive techniques for Mum! I also wished we'd done a pre- and post-summer vacation video, as this would have shown Mum just how badly his speech had regressed.

So, the lesson to be learned here is that parents are not doing their babies *any* favors by giving in to their demands for a bottle— stay firm! Just as with ditching the dummy, you can expect a day or two of tears, but you'll be amazed at how quickly children adapt to change if you make it clear that the bottle is gone for good and that they will only be using a sippy cup from now on.

# WHAT TO DO IF YOUR TWINS HAVE DELAYED LANGUAGE

You may or may not know that twins are at higher risk of speech and language delay than singletons. There are a number of reasons for this but the main ones stem from being premature or having a low birth weight, or possibly because parents don't have as many opportunities to spend one-on-one time with each twin. So, what can you do to help? Try the following ideas.

Find as much time as possible for each twin to have your undivided attention—for example, during nappy changing, or consider bathing them separately from time to time, occasionally having separate bedtime stories, allowing one parent and one twin a head start on a walk, and so on.

Be aware that you are your children's best resource when it comes to learning language, and the more time they have with you, the better. Remember to spend 10 minutes of Special Time every day with each child independently, or at least as often as you can. This will provide an opportunity for each child to practice and improve their communication skills.

You will have to be even more committed to using the Say What You See technique, ensuring that each twin knows that you are commenting on their play and not their sibling's. Remember to back up what you say with signs.

Read to each twin separately. Reading is a fantastic way to encourage language development in all children.

When you are chatting with your twins, make sure there is an equal balance in the conversation—be aware of turn-taking, ensuring that one twin is not dominating the conversation or your time! Allow each twin time to speak, saying, "Gabriel's turn, Alice's turn."

Be aware of your twins talking in their own language—twin language, otherwise known as diglossia. This is very common: One study suggested that twin language occurs in 40 percent of twin pairs.[4]

Twin language usually develops as a result of twins being so in tune with each other that they copy each other's words, even when these attempts at words are incorrect. For example, one twin attempts to say "thank you" by saying "agoo" and before long they are both using "agoo," giving the impression that they have created their own unique language. Remember to always model back the correct version of the word for the child; for example, "Thank you. Well done, you said 'thank you.'" If you are worried, act quickly and get in contact with your local SLP.

## WHAT TO DO IF YOUR CHILD DOESN'T SEEM TO LISTEN TO A WORD YOU SAY

You might be thinking, "What's listening got to do with language development?" Well, I could write an entire book on this topic alone. But in a nutshell, if you can't listen for language, you can't learn language. Many children have to learn how to listen for language and then to integrate their listening skills with their attention skills so that they can "listen and do" at the same time. Let me give you some examples.

Learning to listen in a nursery or preschool setting when there's a lot going on can be tricky for little ones. Think about how different the home and nursery school settings are for some children—moving from a home where Mum might be alone with the little one and her day is navigated around the child's needs and wants to a busy nursery environment where there is a room full of bustling children with just one or two adults around. Your child has to be able to listen selectively, and this requires an immense amount of readjustment.

Even in the relative quiet of home, for many parents, it can feel like our children don't listen to us! Have you ever felt like you're talking to a brick wall? You're calling your child's name, but they're so heavily engrossed in their activity that they haven't even noticed you're speaking to them. They're not listening and therefore not responding. "Yasmin. It's tidy-up time!" No response. "Yasmin. Train game is finished now." Nothing. "YASMIN. NO MORE TRAINS. IT'S TIME TO GET AMI FROM SCHOOL." Nothing. You might have to physically go to your child and touch them, distracting them from their game, getting down to their level, and then saying what you need to say, "The game has finished. Now it's tidy-up time, and let's get in the car to get Ami."

This scenario is not uncommon. In fact, every child developmentally goes through a stage where it appears that they aren't listening to you, and for some children who have delayed attention and listening skills, this stage may go on for much longer.

What follows is the typical developmental pattern to learning to listen and react to stimulus (including you the parent or caregiver!) in a child's environment. These levels were identified in 1978 and revised in 1997, and we as SLPs still use these today.[5] I've included some pointers about what you can do to help at each level if the descriptions sound familiar to you.

## Development of Attention Skills

### Level 1

Extreme Distractibility (0–1 year)

- The child has very fleeting attention that flits constantly from one person to object to event.
- The child can pay fleeting attention, but any new person, event, noise, or smell will be distracting, such as a person walking by or a tree waving in the wind.

**Top Tip Time** How can we help?

- Discover what your child is motivated by and use these motivators in their play; for example, if your child always watches the dog, use the dog in your play: "Look, doggy's eyes, doggy's nose," "Doggy's tail wagging. Stop. Go!" or "Doggy says, 'Woof-woof!'" Or if your baby loves their snuggly blankie, use this when you're playing peekaboo together or hide toys under it for a gone game ("Where's the ball gone? Where's the book gone?"). This will expand your child's ability to focus for longer.

- Get down on their level when you speak, and remember, if your child is only just learning to sit up, all their focus will be going into their ability to sit. Would we be able to concentrate on what someone was saying if we were walking along a tightrope? I think not! So, support your child with cushions so they can use all their energy to focus on their game and your voice.

- You should start reading books to your child when they are babies. Start with repetitive board books and graduate to longer books and stories. Really discover which books your baby likes the best. They'll have favorites at an early age—just like we do!

## Level 2

Single-Channeled Attention (1–2 years)

- "Single-channeled attention" means your child can only focus on one thing at one time, meaning, at this level your child can only concentrate on a motivating task of their own choosing and cannot listen for language at the same time.

- The child must learn to ignore any outside stimulation to be able organize their own thoughts as they play in order to concentrate. For example, while playing with the shape sorter, they wouldn't be able to listen to an adult giving instructions at the same time as trying to push the block into the box. The adult's language interferes with their ability to focus.

- If an older child's attention is functioning at this level, they can sometimes appear rude or obstinate. The reality is, they have to shut you out in order to be able to focus.

**Top Tip Time** **How can we help?**

- We have spoken a lot about the Say What You See technique—putting your child's thought to word as they play. Continue to do this at the right level for your child (single words if your child isn't speaking yet, two or three words if your child is speaking in a few single words, and so on).

- Remember to give your child time to complete their activity; pause and then repeat the phrase after your child has completed the task. For example, with the shape sorter, say, "Turn. Turn. Push. Push!" knowing that these words won't necessarily be retained, but then when the shape has been sorted, and your child looks to you for praise, say, "Hooray. Bye-bye block. Again? One more block?"

- If you are giving an instruction from a distance, for instance, "Tidy-up time. All finished!," then gain your child's attention by going up close, getting down on their level, calling their name, and touching their arm before you speak. This will ensure that they've heard your instruction.

## Level 3

Attention remains single channeled but can be shifted with adult support (2–3 years)

- Level 3 is almost the same as Level 2; a child cannot attend to auditory and visual stimuli at the same time and therefore cannot follow adult instructions while they are playing.

- During this stage, they are starting to learn how to shift their focus from the adult to the task in hand, but the child must learn how to stop their play to attend, listen to the language, then shift their attention back to their activity. This is much easier with adult help.

**Top Tip Time** **How can we help?**

- As we learned in Level 2, gentle physical prompts and then the spoken language will help your child listen to, focus, and retain the spoken language they hear.

- Practice some turn-taking games. My favorites are
  - » building towers. Take turns building a tower, increasing the height of the tower as your child's attention improves. Let your child knock it down as a reward.
  - » rolling a ball or a car to and fro.
- Also, try "ready, steady, go" games with bubbles or cars. Emphasize the "go" and encourage your child to wait for the go cue before you blow the bubbles or push the car. Extend the length of time between the "ready, steady" and the "go" over time so your child has to wait and listen for longer. Always try to gain eye contact with your child during these activities.
- Hide a noisy toy. I use a windup toy or a musical toy and partially hide it; for instance, on a shelf or half behind a cushion so it can still be seen. Say, "Ssshhh, where's your music box?" So they are cued in to listen, then act to find it. Progress to completely hiding the toy so your child has to rely solely on their listening skills.

## Level 4

Single channeled but more easily controlled by the child (3–4 years)

- Your child is now able to voluntarily alternate their full attention, by both looking and listening, between the adult and their activity. A child will automatically look when the adult speaks and then shift their attention back to their task from the speaker.
- However, your child still has to alternate their full attention between a speaker and a task, but they can do this spontaneously, without verbal reminders to focus and refocus.

**Top Tip Time** How can we help?

- Call your child's name, tell them it's time to listen, and, if possible, use a visual cue like this: "Kallum, listen to Mummy.

It's time to go to school [showing a picture of school]."

- While your child is cutting or coloring, tell them to carry on working while listening to you tell them what the plans for the day are, for example.

## Level 5

Learning to have integrated attention (otherwise known as dual-channeled attention) for short bursts of time (4–5 years)

- The child now has dual-channeled attention. They can understand a verbal instruction related to the task they're undertaking without interrupting what they are doing to look at the speaker.
- Their attention span may still be quite short.
- They can be taught in a group and therefore they should be able to listen and attend for short periods of time at school.

**Top Tip Time** **How can we help?**

- Try "One More Turn." When you can sense that your child is losing their focus on a particular task, use the phrase "one more turn" and then allow the activity to end. Once your child has completed the turn give lots of praise and let them go off to play. By doing this, your child will learn to focus for slightly longer.

**Top Tip Time** **How can we help?**

We, the adults, have to modify the way we give information to some children so they have the best chance of listening, retaining, and learning information. Here are some ideas to help.

- Verbal information should be given in short, easy-to-understand chunks. Pause between each chunk to allow your child to process the information.
- Try the following good-listening visual prompts to help engage children in a busy setting. These are

> » a picture of an ear that represents "It's time to listen,"
> » a picture of "sh" meaning, "Try and keep quiet so you can listen," and
> » a picture of eyes meaning, "Try to look at the person who is speaking."

These could be added as real icons if needed.

- The social thinking resources are also great. They encourage "whole-body listening" so that if a child isn't looking at the speaker, you would say, "Listen with your eyes." If a child is fiddling with another child's hair, you say, "Listen with your hands," and so forth. I have even heard an adult say to a child wriggling on their bottom, "Listen with your bottom." Ha! It's important to remember that the social communication and interaction skills of a child with autism are different from—and not lesser than—those of a neurotypical child. Social skills should be taught using "double empathy" (first documented by Dr. Damian Milton), in which each group has an understanding and acceptance of the way the other group communicates.

- Using larger-than-normal gestures and facial expressions will keep your child focused on you. And remember parentese? Research tells us that singsongy voices are more attractive for young children to listen to than flat, monotone voices.

- If it looks like your child hasn't listened or understood, ask them if they want you to repeat the instruction again. Ultimately, your child needs to be encouraged to spontaneously ask if they need information to be repeated. I was delighted when I recently said to a child, "I haven't seen you in yonks and yonks!" and she said, "What is yonks?" Fabulous! Asking for clarification is completely brilliant.

- Encourage your child to look at you before you give any information. Say their name before speaking so that they know you are talking to them.

- In increments, build up the length of time your child needs to listen.

- Break down tasks into steps and encourage your child to do the last step and then the last two steps. This is called backward chaining, and it's a very good way to keep your child focused for longer.

- Use a visual timer—this helps children know how long they have to focus until the activity is finished and they can have a break.

- You know those busy environments where walls are filled with pictures, toys are stacked up all around, and noisy children are everywhere? Well, those sorts of environments make it really tricky for some children to filter out the unwanted stimuli and focus on the important ones. We talk about "arousal-free" settings being the best for our children, but this is far easier said than done!

- Use a visual timetable, which is a set of pictures mapping out the child's day, to help remind the child of the sequence of the day's activities. The child can therefore try to understand what is happening and when a break such as lunch time or snack time is coming.

- Ensure there are frequent breaks throughout your child's day. Movement breaks are especially important for children who are struggling to listen. Moving boosts serotonin, the feel-good hormone, so doing regular movement breaks is a win-win for all. Here are some examples of various movement breaks to try.

  » "Wake up, shake up": a set of gross and fine motor exercises or dance moves to wake up your child's brain and body. Many nursery school settings use the GoNoodle app for this.

  » Clap patterns for call and response: You clap and your child repeats; simple to do and very effective.

  » Offer fidget toys, which have become popular for movement breaks; spinning toys, spinners, poppits, simple dimples, pop tubes, squishies, stress balls, and I have even seen children playing with Blu Tack to help them to focus. Don't allow your child to become dependent on fidgets. Only allow them to have it for a short time (5 to 10 minutes).

» Yoga or stretching breaks: Push your hands together (as if you are praying), hold the fingers on both hands together and pull your fingers apart, hug yourself firmly, and do 3, 2, 1, blast-off, reaching up to the sky when you blast!

» Take turns pretending to be an animal and then copy each other.

» Play catching bubbles.

» Do an obstacle course.

» Try mindfulness breaks where you can practice breathing. First, listen to silence. This can be difficult for some children. Then encourage your child to use their imagination. Close your eyes and imagine you're walking on a beach and feel the sea and sand tickling your toes. Or you're in a pretty garden with lots of flowers and are smelling all the flowers while you walk on the grass.

» Take a comedy break. Tell a joke or watch a couple of funny videos. This will certainly get your brain and body moving!

» Encourage the two hemispheres of the brain to talk to each other by one side of your body doing something different from the other side; for example, pat your head with one hand and rub your tummy with the other, or cross one hand over to the other side of your body by patting your right knee with your left hand and vice versa.

• If your child really struggles to stay seated, do some chair-obics: Squeeze your hands together into a praying shape; hug and squeeze yourself; reach to the sky, then reach over to the right with your left hand and over to the left with your right hand; pat your hands under your bottom and lift your body up; push your knees down so that your feet push firmly into the floor and raise your shoulders up.

• Implement a sensory diet: This isn't diet-related, it's a set of exercises, usually designed by an occupational therapist (OT) trained in sensory integration, that encourage the child to process a number of different sensory stimuli and integrate the senses at the same time.

## WHAT TO DO IF YOUR CHILD STUTTERS

Learning to talk, like learning to walk, is never a completely smooth journey, and it does not happen overnight. Young children often stop, pause, start again, and stumble over words when they are learning to talk. Not even adults have perfectly smooth speech. We often find ourselves getting stuck or stumbling over our words.

Between the ages of 2 and 5, it is normal for a child to repeat words and phrases and to hesitate with "umms" and "errrs" when they are trying to figure out what they want to say. These are known as word-finding difficulties.

However, about 5 in every 100 children stutter for a time when learning to talk. They experience sound or word repetitions: for example, "sh sh sh shop" (known as part or whole-word repetition), or they might stretch out a sound—for instance, "shhhhhop" (called elongation)—or try to say a word without anything coming out of their mouth (known as a block). In approximately 75 percent of these cases, the stutter will resolve, but it should always be handled very carefully, especially if the stutter has been present for longer than six months or if there is a family history of stuttering.

Many children find it easier to talk fluently as they get older. Others continue to find talking difficult, often getting stuck and feeling as if they can't talk properly. Whatever the situation, I would advise that it is always better to get them some help.

### What is stuttering?

A child is thought to be stuttering when they

- put extra effort into saying words,
- talk in a tense or jerky style,

- have trouble getting started, so no sound comes out,
- stretch out words—for instance, "I want a sssstory,"
- repeat the first sound of a word or part of a word—for example, "m . . . m . . . mummy" or "mum mum mum mummy," and/or
- stop and give up trying to speak.

## How is fluency affected?

Stuttering may come and go. The child's speech may be fluent for several days or weeks, then the speaking may become difficult again. Fluency can be affected by

- an increase in complexity of language (it's as if the child's brain is thinking too quickly for their mouth),
- growth spurts, which lead to clumsy movements in general, after which the body tends to readjust and right itself,
- difficult or unusual situations at home or at nursery school; busy times when turn-taking in talking; exciting or rushed moments,
- talking to different and new people—adults or children, family or strangers, or
- how the child is feeling—unwell, tired, anxious, excited, or confident.

## What can help stuttering?

If your child has a stutter, consult an SLP as soon as possible. The SLP is likely to give you the following advice.

- Slow your own rate of speech to make it easier for your child to follow what you are saying and to help them to feel less rushed. They will, hopefully, copy you and slow down, too. This can be more helpful and less intrusive than telling them to "slow down," "start again," or "take a deep breath."
- Use the same sort of sentences your child does—keep them short and simple.

- It may help to pause for one second before you answer or ask a question. This is for two reasons—first, taking a pause will slow down the rate of the conversation, and second, your child might copy you and learn to take a pause before they answer a question, giving them a split second of extra thinking time to put their thoughts together and form a sentence.

- Show your child you are interested in *what they are talking about* rather than *how they are talking*. Get down to their level and look at them so that they know you are interested.

- Reduce the number of questions you ask—conversation should not be an interrogation!

- Have a Special Time every day—aim for one 10-minute slot per day when your child is not talking over others and the attention is wholly on them. Spend time together playing what your child wants to play and talking about what they want to talk about—this will ensure a relaxed, unrushed environment. Don't forget to praise them when they say things smoothly and for the efforts they make—this will boost their confidence.

The British Stammering Association has kindly given me permission to reproduce this advice on what can help stuttering (also known as stammering). For more help and support, contact your local SLP immediately and/or the National Stuttering Association (westutter.org).

## WHAT TO DO IF YOUR BILINGUAL HOME AFFECTS SPEECH DEVELOPMENT

My neighborhood is very multicultural and it is common for me to see a child who lives in a home where one or even two foreign languages are spoken, and who goes to an English-speaking school, so that the child is exposed to two or three different languages. This is something that SLPs embrace rather than worry about. Imagine the long-term advantages this child will have if they can speak three languages fluently. Wowzers!

Until quite recently, experts thought that bringing up a child in a bilingual home could cause language confusion, which would lead to a delay in speech development.

However, research now tells us to encourage parents to make the most of young children's spongelike knack for acquiring language and revel in their ability to switch between languages, potentially boosting the speed at which the brain works. And there are other benefits, too. Over the past decade, Ellen Bialystok, a research professor of psychology at York University in Toronto, has established that bilingual children develop crucial skills in addition to their double vocabularies, learning different ways to solve logic problems or to handle multitasking—skills that are often considered part of the brain's so-called executive function.

However, that doesn't mean that raising a bilingual or trilingual child is easy—it can be confusing and worrying for parents, and many are desperate for more information about how to juggle all the languages their child is exposed to. I share here my best strategies for nurturing a happy, confident, and chatty bilingual child.

- The general rule is "one place, one language" and, if this is not possible, then "one person, one language." This is in an ideal world and, in reality, a lot of families switch from one language to another fairly frequently throughout the day and so do the children. If this is the case, try to ensure you don't mix two languages in one sentence, conversation, or activity; it is definitely better to keep the languages apart if possible.

- Try to speak only one language at a time—so when reading a book, *don't* say "ball" in English and then "bola" in Spanish, for example. Read the whole thing through in English and then again in Spanish. During mealtimes, try to stick to one language and not switch between two. This is not always possible, but we're talking about an ideal world!

- If your child is going to be bilingual, they need a high level of exposure to two languages over a long period of time.

All the same games and activities to encourage language development—nursery rhymes, books, play, discussions, word games, and daily language-rich activities such as visits to the park or supermarket—should be carried out in both languages.

- It's very common for a child to go through a silent period, which can last a few months, when they are first immersed in a setting where a language different from their mother tongue is spoken. This is normal and allows the child an opportunity to hear and understand the language before they start to speak it. If this silent period lasts longer than four months, speak to an SLP for advice.

- It is normal for a child to refuse to speak in a particular language for a short time and only answer in another language, and your child may even tell you that they hate talking in a particular language. Continue as you always have done—this is just a phase and it will pass. Remember—the long-term benefits far surpass periodic disagreements.

## Myth-busting

There are a couple of myths about raising bilingual children that should be laid to rest.

### Myth: Language delays in a child's mother tongue are caused by learning a second language

This is not true. Learning a second language neither increases nor decreases the chances of having a language delay, and delays in learning language are just as common in monolingual children as they are in a bilingual community. If your child is thought to have a speech or language problem, or an additional need of some sort, *don't* stop speaking to them in the language in which you have always spoken to them—this will only hinder their language development. It's amazing how many parents do this or are told to do this, thinking that if there is only one language, the child will learn faster so long as the two languages aren't mixed together in the same conversation. There is no evidence to suggest that this is true. Just to reiterate, no one should ever tell you to give up talking in any language you speak. Being bilingual is not bad for your child, will not hold them back, confuse them or make life difficult for them; on the contrary, the advantages are vast!

## HOW BILINGUALISM SHAPES THE BRAIN

Researchers at the University of Washington compared the electrical brain responses in infants from homes in which one language was spoken (monolingual) with those of infants exposed to two languages at home.[6]

They found that at 6 months, the monolingual infants could discriminate between speech sounds, whether they were uttered in the language they were used to hearing or in another language not spoken in their homes. By 10 to 12 months, however, monolingual babies were no longer detecting sounds in the other language, only in the language they usually heard. The researchers suggest that this represents a process of neural commitment, by which the infant's brain wires itself to understand one language and its sounds.

In contrast, the bilingual infants followed a different developmental trajectory. At 6 to 9 months, they did not detect differences in phonetic sounds in either language, but when they were older—10 to 12 months—they were able to discriminate sounds in both.

"What the study demonstrates is that the variability in bilingual babies' experiences keeps them open," says Dr. Patricia Kuhl, codirector of the Institute for Learning and Brain Sciences at the University of Washington and one of the authors of the study. "It's another piece of evidence that what you experience shapes the brain."

## Myth: It's easier to learn a second language if you stop using your first or home language and concentrate on the new language

This is definitely *not* true. We say that the stronger the first language is, the easier it is to learn a second language, because the child has already been exposed to, and has a grasp of, all the vocabulary and grammatical structures needed to acquire a language. Some families get into muddy waters when they switch to English in order to prepare their child for school. *Please don't do this.* The child can get very confused, not knowing which language is which, so just leave English to school—it'll be so much easier for your child.

If you are worried, instead of speaking to your child in English yourself (particularly if it's broken English), take them to a toddler group, a caregiver, or the house of a friend who speaks English before they start school. An old teacher colleague of mine says it takes about one academic year for a 3- to 4-year-old attending nursery school every morning to be fluent in English if they have not had any exposure to English prior to this.

---

### BILINGUALISM STARTS IN THE WOMB!

Janet Werker, a professor of psychology at the University of British Columbia, studies how babies perceive language and how that shapes their learning. Even in the womb, she says, babies are exposed to the rhythms and sounds of language, and newborns have been shown to prefer languages that are rhythmically similar to the one they've heard during fetal development.

In one recent study, Dr. Werker and her collaborators showed that babies born to bilingual mothers not only prefer both of those languages over others but are also able to register that the two languages are different.

---

# WHAT TO DO IF YOUR CHILD HAS GLUE EAR, OR OTITIS MEDIA WITH EFFUSION (OME)

Otitis media with effusion (OME) is a temporary hearing problem in which the middle ear fills up with fluid instead of air, which muffles sound. Having OME is rather like trying to hear while wearing a huge pair of earmuffs. OME can fluctuate, but during a "stuffy" phase, a child can't hear language and speech sounds consistently, which means they can fall behind and/or pick up bad speech-sound habits.

OME is very common in young children because they do not have robust immune systems and tend to catch many of the bugs going around, and they may be prone to congestion from lots of coughs, colds, ear infections, or allergies such as hay fever. When a child gets stuffed up, so does the small tube that connects the nasal cavity to the middle ear, consequently filling the middle ear.

The incidence levels of OME peak from about 2 to 6 years of age. In the 2- to 5-year age range 15 to 20 percent of children will have OME at any time. The prevalence in children older than this falls to less than 5 percent by age 7. In the vast majority of cases, OME will not persist beyond early childhood.[7]

## Detecting OME

Your child may have otitis media with effusion (OME) if

- they get lots of colds,
- they do not hear so well—for instance, if they turn up the volume on the TV frequently—or say "What?" or "Uh?" a lot,
- their behavior deteriorates,
- they become quieter than usual,
- their concentration is poor,
- they find listening with background noise difficult,
- they're unable to hear the differences between some speech sounds, which can affect pronunciation,

- they tune out because listening is hard work and, therefore, they miss information, and/or
- they appear clumsy and have poor balance. (My daughter, Jess, weirdly started falling over a lot at the age of 16 months, and my mum insisted I take her to the doctor. I felt like a fool, but the doctor took it very seriously, partly because Jess went splat on his office floor, and he sent her to a pediatrician and for a hearing test. Sure enough, she had otitis media with effusion and had to be retested in four months.)

If you are worried that your child may have otitis media with effusion, see your pediatrician, who will look in their ears and possibly refer them for a hearing test. An audiologist is likely to monitor their hearing over a two- to three-month period in most cases. Consultants will often insert a grommet in each ear (a little tube that fits into the child's eardrum in order to drain the fluid) but if the parent prefers, the child will be given hearing aids instead of undergoing an operation.

There are adjustments that you can make to help a child with otitis media with effusion. First, keep background noise to a minimum—turn off the TV, move away from noises when talking to your child, and if you have a busy, bustling home, try to have some quiet times. Also, encourage your child to look at you when you are talking so they can watch your mouth to work out how you are making those tricky speech sounds.

Ensure you have your child's attention before you speak. Keep your voice clear and speak slightly louder than usual, without shouting. Talk to them when they are near you so they have a better chance of hearing you. Be patient and explain things more than you usually would—your child may be mishearing or confusing similar-sounding words. And make sure you spend some one-on-one time with them every day, doing the Top Tip Time activities that follow.

**Top Tip Time** **Otitis media with effusion**

If you know your child has OME, you might like to do some focused work in order to improve their speech and language development.

- Practice lots of listening games. If your child's ears become used to not hearing, even when the hearing improves, you might have to retrain their ears to listen to sounds.

- Focus on phonics (speech sounds) and ensure your child can discriminate one single speech sound from another, then see if they can determine which sound particular words start with. Take a selection of toys, animals, perhaps, and say, "Find an animal that starts with 'b.'"

---

## OME AT NURSERY SCHOOL OR PRESCHOOL

If your child has had an otitis media with effusion diagnosis from your pediatrician, let your child's teachers, caregivers or nursery school workers know, and encourage them to take the following actions.

- Ensure your child is sitting near the speaker during communal times, such as mealtime, carpet time, story time, or song times.

- Check whether your child has heard an instruction by encouraging them to repeat it back prior to carrying it out—for instance, "What did Gill say? She said, 'Everybody stand up, collect your lunch boxes, and line up by the door.'"

- Have a quiet time and practice listening games, as suggested above.

---

## WHAT TO DO IF AN OLDER SIBLING IS AFFECTING YOUR TODDLER'S LANGUAGE DEVELOPMENT

In chapter 8, we considered how the birth of a new baby might affect an older sibling's language, but let's consider other possibilities concerning siblings that might also have an impact.

We've learned that boys need a little extra attention when it comes to certain aspects of learning, so imagine a scenario in which a new baby boy is born into a family where the older sibling—a very articulate, sociable, and confident older sister—rules the roost. We must ensure the younger brother is included and that the amount of time spent in both one-on-one engagement with a parent and with the entire family is balanced. For example, during mealtimes when everybody is telling their news, allow the younger baby to tell their news, too—it might be a load of babble or gibberish, but allow them a chance to get a word in, in order for their language skills to develop.

In some of the families I visit at home, I have noticed that there's a bit of a habit of "parking" a younger baby in a reclining bouncer seat or even a car seat, to the side of what's happening with the older children. Try to include your younger children in as much of the action as possible. Allow them to sit with you as you play together, or use a jumping baby bouncer, which allows them to feel much more included in whatever's going on.

## HOW TO PICK A NURSERY SCHOOL FOR A CHILD WITH LANGUAGE DELAY

One of the (many!) difficult decisions parents are likely to have to make in the early years is choosing a nursery school or caregiver. You are likely to be fraught with guilt and insecurity about going back to work, and the stress of finding the right person to look after your precious little one while you aren't there, and the right setting for their individual needs, is enormous.

Unfortunately, I can't help you make the tricky choice, but having been grilled by lots of friends about what questions to ask and what to look out for in terms of finding a positive speech and communication environment for babies and toddlers, I do have some pointers. Here are my observations and recommendations.

## Nursery schools

- The most important thing in a child's early years is to feel special to many people, but to one or two people in particular, so that they know that *that* person is *their* special person. Who will your child go to when they need a cuddle or when they're upset if you're not there? Ideally, your child will have a key worker with whom they can form a strong bond in this new environment. By 2½ or 3 years of age, a child is more sociable and independent and, therefore, has more confidence to be an independent person in a nursery setting.

  A friend of mine has a little boy who had a hard time settling into his nursery school, even though it had a glowing reputation. When my friend asked what happened when he cried, the manager said the workers looked after him in turns. That didn't allow him to build a strong bond with one adult in particular, which made settling in more difficult. The nursery school told my friend that they waited for a child to find his own key person—but what would happen if every child formed a strong attachment to the same person? This is one of the main ways in which caregivers and nurseries differ—a caregiver has specific children to look after in their home, so they are automatically the child's key person.

  Every nursery school, meanwhile, should have a policy on key workers, and you should definitely ask about it. Will your child be handed to, and collected from, the same person every day? Will your child's key person have an opportunity to spend individual time with them every day to make them feel special and to nurture them? Will your child's key person have a chance to think about and discuss your child with you if there is a problem?

- Ask about the child-to-staff ratio. The American Academy of Pediatrics (AAP) recommends that one adult should have the *primary responsibility* for no more than one baby under 12 months of age in any care setting. Babies need positive, consistent caregivers who learn to recognize their unique cues for hunger, distress and play. This kind of nurturing interaction contributes significantly to an infant's social and emotional growth. For overall infant care, the AAP recommends a child-to-staff ratio of 3:1; then this goes up to 4:1 for 2- to 3-year olds, 5:1 for 3- to 4-year olds, and 6:1 for children ages 4 to 5 years old.

- I'm not a fan of nursery schools that have a baby room and a toddler room, splitting up children of different ages. In terms of boosting speech, it's far better for toddlers and babies to mix, as it creates a more typical family environment. The little ones pick up new words from the older ones, while the older ones learn to tell stories to the younger ones, help them to wash their hands, and generally nurture them, giving them an opportunity to use the language they have been exposed to by their parents. This is called a family group, and it tends to work well for both older and younger children.

- Think about how the layout of the nursery school works— I'm not keen on large, open-plan nurseries because I suspect a child gets far less adult contact in such rooms and, of course, they need an adult to provide them with a model for language. So, look for cozy areas in which your child can be in proximity to an adult who can model language and expand their language skills as they play. A good nursery will also have little adult-free areas. These child-only spaces are designed to encourage confidence at peer level for social and verbal communication.

- I know you should think about people more than toys, but do look at the resources the nursery has. For instance, have the puzzles got all their pieces? Has the toy kitchen got some food in it and a spoon? This is a good indication of whether the profits of the nursery school are coming back to the children or staying with the management.

- When you visit, watch the nursery staff to see how they interact with the children. Ideally, they will be
  - » talking to the children and kneeling down to their level,
  - » using simple language, backed up with signs and gestures,

> » supporting the children's play, not taking over or being passive,

> » helping children extend their play by one level (so that, if your child is playing with the trains, a member of staff will bring another element into the game by saying, for instance, something like, "Toby's come off the track—how can we help him?"), and

> » trying to find out about your child, their likes and dislikes, and what they are motivated by.

- Consider the atmosphere of the nursery—have the staff members created a good atmosphere or does it feel clinical? Are they warm and welcoming? If they don't make an effort in this way when they're trying to win your favor, they're certainly not going to when you've walked out the door.

- The environment should be as visual as possible—ideally there will be lots of artwork by the children up on the walls, pictures on the drawers showing what's inside, and short vocabulary suggestions for the staff to say and repeat visible in each area of the nursery (for instance, "splash"/"pour"/"wash" by the water tray). The story and song time should also be visually supported with props (for example, a story sack with the food that the Very Hungry Caterpillar eats and a selection of objects that represent songs, such as a tractor for singing "Bouncing Up and Down in My Little Red Wagon").

- Ask the staff about the outside-play activities they engage the children in. Ideally, some of these should revolve around learning as well as playing. This is referred to as play-based learning. So, they might have pets to look after, play sorting games in paddling pools where they have to sort items that float or items that don't, do nature hunts, visit a mobile library, and so on. My sister-in-law runs a nursery called Free Rangers that includes a forest school within the nursery, so that, every day, the children have outdoor play-based learning rather than just a breath of fresh air.

- At mealtimes, does the staff eat with the children? This provides a good model for fussy eaters, and a staff member will be able to encourage communication, as mealtimes are one of the most social times of the day.

- How does the staff communicate to you, and what about? Do they provide daily summaries in a nursery school book—ideally filled in by your child's key person—in which, occasionally, some sentences are written in red to show what the next developmental step would be?

## Caregivers

The difference between a caregiver and a nursery school is that with the former a child has a closer contact with, and feels special to, one—and only one—person. And this is one of the reasons people tend to choose nursery schools—they cannot stand the thought of their child becoming too close to another adult. Jess loves our caregiver, and rather than feeling jealous about how attached she is to Lyn, I feel thankful and relieved that I have chosen the best caregiver I could have for her.

When looking for a good caregiver, many of the factors that should inform your choice of nursery school (see previous section) also apply, along with the tips below.

- One thing to be careful about is the number of school and nursery school pickups and drop-offs your caregiver has to do. Will your child be spending much of their day in a car or outside a school gate?
- Find out if the caregiver will take your child to a local toddler group. If so, will they be communicating with them while they are there? A work colleague of mine collected her son for a doctor's appointment from a toddler group that the caregiver took him to most days. She said that many of the caregivers were chatting on their cell phones while the children were playing. You should ask where your child will be going and find out the reputation of that particular place, and visit it, too.

I've covered the basics here. Just don't forget the most important thing—trust your instincts. If you want to feel confident you've made the right choice for you and your toddler, look at many different nursery schools and caregivers in your area with my pointers in mind, and one is bound to stand out to you as being the best fit.

## HOW TO CHOOSE AND GET THE BEST OUT OF STORYBOOKS

Throughout this book I suggest using storybooks to help expand your child's language skills. This is because, besides yourself, books and stories are the ultimate resource for helping your child to develop advanced language skills. There are many reasons for this, and here I have listed a few. Sharing a book regularly with your child

- provides a lovely opportunity to snuggle up, share a moment together, and bond with each other. It gives you an opportunity to hear and watch your child as they communicate,
- helps your child develop better attention and listening skills as they learn to concentrate for the duration of the whole book, while they turn the pages, look at the pictures, and listen to familiar words in increasingly longer sentences,
- develops a child's understanding because looking at the same books over and again allows them to hear a repetition of the same words while looking at corresponding pictures, and the repetition develops and cements their understanding of the words and the narrative,
- helps a child learn new words, hear longer sentences and be exposed to grammatical structures to help develop their expressive language,
- provides an opportunity to work on making choices. Even with a very little baby, ensure you offer a choice of which book they would like to read,

- helps to develop fine motor control, by turning the pages and pointing to the pictures, so encourage your child to do so,
- provides older children with a format with which to retell their own stories,
- helps with many aspects of language development, such as use of tenses, prediction and narrative. Ask your child what happened on the previous page once you have turned it, what might happen next before you turn the page and what might happen at the end. Then ask them to retell the whole story when you've finished,
- encourages your child to get into a daily reading routine or an academic routine that will stand them in good stead for life, and
- expands your child's thought and opens up and enriches their life as they enter a world of dragons, fairy princesses and princes, faraway countries, and other things that are not in their own daily experience.

## Selecting books for your child

Choose books that are suitable for your child's age group. The Top Tip that follows should help you make the right book choices for your child.

### Approximately 0–6 months

Very young babies love being snuggled and enjoy listening to the sound of a parent's voice and looking at pictures in high contrast (for instance, pictures in black-and-white or black-and-yellow), especially pictures of faces.

Then they move on to board books with simple but bold pictures and one or two words per page. Encourage your child to turn the pages by lifting one page up slightly with your right hand. Remember to always offer a choice of book; at this age, your child will reach for the one they want.

Try books with familiar songs in them and cloth books, so that your child can give them a good chew.

## Approximately 6–12 months

Try fairly short books—about one sentence per page or less—with bright colors and sturdy pages. And if there's a repetitive line, even better. Try *Brown Bear, Brown Bear, What Do You See?* by Bill Martin Jr. and Eric Carle or *Dear Zoo* by Rod Campbell. Try bath books and noisy books and also make a family book (an album) yourself with all your child's favorite people in it.

## Approximately 12–18 months

At this age, children still enjoy repetition, so I often add a repetitive line when there isn't one (for example, when reading *Where's Spot?*, I will add the line "Where's Spot?" each time I turn the page). Also, why not try a book with a rhythm or rhyme? Children will be more interested in the pictures than the story. Lift-the-flap books are good, but pop-up books are not so great because all the pictures get ripped out!

If possible, sit so that your child can see your face and the book, so they can watch your mouth move. Better still, if you can use your hands as you are talking, it'll really help the book to come alive—you'll need a cookbook stand! My favorite books for this age group include *Goodnight Moon* by Margaret Wise Brown and Clement Hurd, *Pip and Posy: The Big Balloon* by Axel Scheffler, *The Going to Bed Book* by Sandra Boynton, and *Where's Spot?* by Eric Hill.

## Approximately 18–24 months

Children of this age group still like the types of books previously listed, but they are beginning to like a story line running though. My favorite books for this age group include *The Tiger Who Came to Tea* by Judith Kerr, *We're Going on a Bear Hunt* by Michael Rosen and Helen Oxenbury, *Handa's Surprise* by Eileen Browne, *The Very Hungry Caterpillar* by Eric Carle, and *Chocolate Mousse for Greedy Goose* by Julia Donaldson and Nick Sharratt.

Also seek out books that will extend your child's vocabulary, such as DK's *Hide and Seek First Words* or *The Baby's Catalogue* by Janet and Allan Ahlberg.

## Approximately 2–3 years

When choosing books for 2- to 3-year-olds, look for those with a basic story supported by quite busy pictures so that, if your child doesn't understand the words, they can see the pictures. Children love the detail in the pictures and love it when you point something out that they haven't yet noticed. A child will like a book that means something. For example, the mother of a friend of mine died, and when she broke the news to her son, she told him that her mother was now a star, and the book *How to Catch a Star* by Oliver Jeffers then went down really well.

Other books that are great for this age group include the *The Gruffalo* and *The Gruffalo's Child* by Julia Donaldson and Axel Scheffler, *Who Sank the Boat?* by Pamela Allen, *Where's Waldo?* by Martin Handford, and the My Big Wimmelbooks series. And for extending vocabulary, try *Richard Scarry's Best First Book Ever!*

## Approximately 3–4 years

At this age, a child likes a good story, perhaps a fairy tale with longer paragraphs—probably five sentences or more per page. They also love humor and expanding their thought and imagination. Good books for this age group include *The Gingerbread Man* by Karen Schmidt, *Rumble in the Jungle* by Giles Andreae and David Wojtowycz, *Charlie Cook's Favorite Book* and *A Squash and a Squeeze* by Julia Donaldson and Axel Scheffler, *Q Pootle 5* by Nick Butterworth, *Mixed-Up Fairy Tales* by Hilary Robinson and Nick Sharratt, and *The Astonishing Secret of Awesome Man* by Michael Chabon and Jake Parker.

Another thing to try at this age is picture books without words to help your child to retell the story by themselves. You could try *Window* by Jeannie Baker or *Hug* by Jez Alborough.

# WHAT TO DO IF YOUR CHILD WANTS TO WATCH A SCREEN AT MEALTIME

You may wonder why I am even mentioning eating in a book that's all about talking, but the fact of the matter is, mealtimes are one of the most sociable times of the day, and it's important that we make the most of them, getting good habits established as early as we possibly can! Before you know it, your child will be associating food with fun and with an opportunity to share stories about their day, laughing and connecting with family over some delicious flavors and aromas that everyone is enjoying! It is perhaps a sign of our busy and disrupted times that sitting down at a table to eat together is a dying tradition and one I am passionate about reviving.

As a speech pathologist, I have an additional qualification to assess eating and drinking issues in children, and I am often called in by schools or families to help children who are unable to eat without a tablet or screen perched beside their plate. The root cause might be that parents have struggled to get their child to eat when that little one was being weaned, so they start using a screen as some sort of distraction while they shovel food in, or that they simply don't have time to sit with their child at every mealtime (believe me, I get it!) so they give their child a screen for company while they go on doing the dishes or preparing supper. Either way, once a screen is involved, the habit often sticks, and then you have a child who refuses to eat without a screen—and mealtimes have become a digital battleground. Argh!

If this sounds familiar to you—or you can see yourself heading down that road—here is what to do.

**Top Tip Time** **Creating Sociable Mealtimes**

To keep a meal sociable, try to eat something alongside your baby so they are exposed to the range of foods you eat. Be confident and enjoy watching them as they devour your culinary delights! Of course, I realize that we can't all sit down for dinner with our children at 5:00 PM every day, but try to do it when you can, even if it's just lunch or supper on the weekends because you are working during the week. And you can make up for it by making it a really fun and sociable mealtime!

Setting the scene for mealtimes is important, so try to have a routine in place for meals, just as you have an established bedtime routine.

## 6 MONTHS

Be sure to sit your baby in a high chair in which they are well supported—they shouldn't be wobbling around. If they are, stuff a towel down the side for a snugger fit. Your baby's feet should also be flat on a surface; if their legs are dangling, then it'll feel to them as if they are sitting on a gym ball as they eat (i.e., very, very unsteady). Don't feed your child in a recliner seat—it's tricky for babies to control their head movements, and depending on the level of the recline, the food can rush to the back of their mouths too quickly to swallow it and can result in coughing and spluttering.

## 12–18 MONTHS

Let's get our little ones chatting with a few food-related words and sounds and get those mouth muscles moving at the same time! You can do this by encouraging babbling during mealtimes. For example, say, "Mmm," when your child is eating to encourage lip closure (you can't make this sound without closing your lips), and say "b-b-b-banana," "yum-yum," or "mmmore."

Certain foods are more fun than others—spaghetti is a great example! There is a muscle that completely encircles lips, known as the orbicularis oris, which allows you to purse your lips into a circle to say "ooo" and "sh" among other sounds, and also to make raspberry noises and kiss! If this muscle is strengthened, your baby's sounds will be easier to achieve and more clearly artic-ulated. My friend's baby, Cecilie, was sucking up spaghetti at the age of 9 months, and she loved it so much it made her squeal with laughter—a fantastic exercise for the lips and great fun, as every-one else at the table will be laughing and joining in, too!

Don't feel put off from going to restaurants or cafés because you have a little one—think of these excursions as part of their education! It's a chance to try new things in a new environment, likely pushing your boundaries as well as theirs. I always remem-ber going for lunch with my mother-in-law just a week after I had started weaning Jess when she was 6 months old. I was having a salad with a chunk of pineapple that Jess reached for and I willing-ly gave it to her to suck and practice biting on. She then wanted the lemon from my drink and, much to the horror of my mother-in-law, I gave it to her, peel and all, after taking out the seeds. Sure enough, she loved it!

### Food play games to try

*Warning!* If you have a fussy eater, you might have to accept that not all the games revolve around "healthy" food but, trust me, a bit of chocolate mousse won't hurt them, and if it gets them in-terested in eating, who cares? These games are aimed at little ones from 8 to 18 months.

- Put on an apron and practice painting with jam—encourage your baby to lick their fingers, but do not force them.
- Try drawing with a tube of icing.
- Help your baby make a mask out of a paper plate by sticking on dried pasta shapes for the eyes, nose, and mouth. The tri-color pasta (that is, orange, green, and white pasta) works well for this game.
- Try vegetable stamping by cutting interesting shapes in potatoes, carrots or other hard vegetables, dipping them in paint, and printing them on paper.
- Try painting with broccoli sticks or carrots.

- Put sprinkles on buttered bread to make a pretty pattern.
- My personal favorite game is hiding toy animals or cars in jelly or cereal. Children are always delighted to find their dinosaurs or doggies buried in squishy jelly.

**Top Tip Time** Tongue

Having a strong tongue will help your little one move the food around their mouth to chew it and to articulate clear and crisp speech sounds. Have a go at the following licking games and tongue exercises.

- Plant a bit of yogurt on each corner and on the top and the bottom of your baby's lips. Encourage them to lick it off—this is probably best done in a mirror so that they can see what they're doing.
- Put some chocolate sprinkles at the bottom of a ramekin and encourage your baby to lick down to taste them.
- Encourage your child to lick their lips before you wipe their messy mouth.
- Make funny faces in the mirror using your tongue.
- Make up a story about Mr. Tongue! It goes something like this: "Mr. Tongue wakes up one morning and comes out of his house [your mouth]. He decides to have a good stretch right up to the sky [move your tongue upward]. And then down to the ground [move your tongue downward]. And then he sees a dog wagging his tail and he tries to copy [move tongue from side to side]," and so on.
- I also love the song "The Little Green Frog." The key feature is that you must poke out your tongue as you sing and it's great fun for you and baby!

So, all that fabulous foody floor and face mess is well worth it! The wonderful social interactions you have at mealtimes, and opportunities to develop speech and language skills will set your tiny talker up for expanding their language in the months and years to come.

# WHAT TO DO IF YOU THINK YOUR CHILD MIGHT BE AUTISTIC

I see hundreds of children in my clinic every year for speech and language therapy, and almost every single one of their parents asks me if I think their child has autism. The reason being that virtually every child in the world, at one time in their life through to adulthood, will display one or two and perhaps even a few characteristics that are associated with autism. All it takes is for your baby to seemingly avoid eye contact for a few days, your toddler to jump up and flap their hands in excitement, or your preschooler to be obsessed with dinosaurs, and speculation sweeps in.

And, unlike many childhood conditions, syndromes, or structural abnormalities, there is no neonatal test to diagnose autism. Cue more worry. After all, isn't that a parent's job?

More than likely there won't be any cause for concern and those tots who had seemed disengaged, different, or quirky at times quickly become the most sociable children you know. But with the incidence rates of autism forever increasing and early diagnosis and intervention thought to be of paramount importance, parents need to be aware of the symptoms so they can detect, intervene, and adapt to their child's needs as early as possible (adaptations to the parents' communication style and the child's environment are thought to have the biggest impact on a young child's development).

Autism assessment is one component of my day job—I am a specialist at diagnosing autism in under-fives. So, here I'll share as much of my expertise as possible—and metaphorically "hold your hand" as you start to work out what you can do to help.

## What is autism?

In a nutshell, autism is classified as a social communication disorder ("disorder" meaning the development is deviating from what might be considered "typical"). More recently, there is a move toward "autistic spectrum condition" as a label rather than "autistic spectrum disorder," because "disorder" suggests the child has a disability, and we as parents and professionals are moving away from what is considered to be negative terminology when talking about autism, ensuring autism is seen as a difference and not a disadvantage. So, a child with autism's social interaction and social communication skills may look slightly different from that of a child without autism, and features of restrictive and repetitive patterns of interests and behaviors will be evident. This is why it's easier to diagnose autism after 18 months of age, when the differences in children's social interaction skills become more apparent.

You may also have heard of sensory processing or sensory integration difficulties. These are very common in children with autism, too, and consequently, children may experience difficulties in learning about the world through their senses. This is explained in the "What to do if your child doesn't seem to listen to a word you say" section (see page 242).

For a child (or adult) to receive a diagnosis of autism, they must have traits in two areas: social communication and interaction, and restrictive and repetitive patterns of behavior and interests. This is known as the "dyad of impairment," and it correlates with the diagnostic criteria for autism within the DSM-5 (Diagnostic and Statistical Manual of Mental Disorders 5).

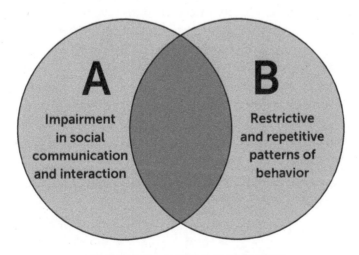

**DIAGNOSTIC CRITERIA FOR AUTISM**

# THE NEURODIVERSITY PARADIGM

The neurodiversity paradigm encourages a new and more inclusive way of looking at and thinking about autism. "Neurodiversity" is a relatively new term but signals an important shift in how autism is viewed, driven by autistic individuals themselves speaking out. Because of their advocacy, our understanding of autism has deepened. Take, for example, the language we speech pathologists have been using in our therapy rooms when working with children who have autism. I cringe when I think how we previously focused on children's "disorder," "ability," or "inability." And I'm appalled that when we spoke to parents, we'd talk about goals that would target "normalizing" their autistic child's social skills or reducing restrictive and repetitive thoughts or behaviors so that they could "fit in."

This outdated and reductive way of thinking leads children to mask their true communication style as they try to copy what they perceive to be "normal." It causes stress and anxiety and other mental health concerns, and it instills in a child at a young age the idea that being different is bad, knocking down their confidence for life.

Instead, with the neurodiversity paradigm, we are homing in on the child's environment to make it easier for them to feel calm, focused, and secure—the optimal state for learning. The supporting adults are encouraged to follow the child's lead in play, to use visual supports instead of complex verbal instructions, and to attempt to understand what motivates them. Furthermore, we encourage autistic children to map out their own needs—for instance, to choose when they need a sensory break or indicate whether they would like to communicate with a device instead of verbally. We are moving away from the idea that neurodivergent individuals need to be "normalized" and instead, we are focusing on their ability to shine and thrive in their own unique and wonderful way!

# Traits of autism in young children

So what does autism look like for a little one? It won't surprise you to learn that autism affects children in many ways and every child diagnosed with autism has their own unique profile. Here are a few common features of autism in children between 1 and 4 years old. (NOTE: This is by no means an exhaustive list.)

## Social communication and social interaction features in children with autism

- Not greeting others or not noticing when people walk into a room
- Little interest in playing with, talking to, or showing things to others
- Having delayed language development. Perhaps consistently pulling parents to what they want or placing your hand on something they want—for example, to open a tube of bubbles, but not attempting a word, sound, or gesture to enhance their ability to express themselves.
- Limited consistent attempts at single words and often evidence of jargon (using utterances that have no meaning and sound like gibberish)
- Repetitive and/or rigid language skills—for example, reciting numbers, songs, or parts of a favorite TV show. You may also hear echolalia—when a child repeats exactly what they've just heard rather than answering. This may also occur when a child incorrectly generalizes a learned phrase in a number of different situations; for example, they might say, "Cookie, please" when they are looking at an apple. Therefore, "cookie, please" means I am hungry or I want that apple, even though they are looking at an apple when they feel hungry.
- Not pointing or using other gestures such as "bye-bye," or "up" when they want to be lifted up
- Difficulty copying, both verbally and in play routines

- Difficulty copying or understanding facial expressions
- Reduced eye contact with others or perhaps only looking very fleetingly
- Not responding or engaging when someone tries to play interactively with them. They are content to be in their own world, with a strong preference for child-initiated play.

## Restrictive and repetitive behaviors typical in children with autism

- Narrow interests, maybe even becoming obsessed by something—for example, watching the machine spinning around or the wheels spinning on a toy car. Older children may have a special interest in dinosaurs, trains, horses, dogs, cats, other animals, numbers, the solar system, or best friends.
- Does the same routines with repetitive play patterns—for example, wanting the same song or book over and over again
- Not understanding someone else's point of view, or that someone else's mind works differently than their own (this is known as "theory of mind"); for example, when a parent folds a duvet back on a bed and points to the bed, they are expecting the child to get into the bed. "Mind-blindness" (integral for predicting and interpreting other people's behaviors) is not understanding that *you* have a different brain and heart from mine and that my brain thinks thoughts and my heart feels feelings in a different way from yours.
- Playing the same game the same way every time or wanting the same phrases in books read over and over again—a desire for sameness—and tuning in to the intonation patterns of the words rather than the meaning of the individual words and sentences
- Not keen on daily transitions—for instance, moving from watching TV in the den to eating breakfast in the kitchen or playing outside to coming inside. They're not keen when routines change and they prefer things to be predictable, perhaps insisting on sameness—the same route, same greeting, or same food every day.

- Might be obsessed with an object and carry it around with them—for example, a straw or a figurine
- Preferring to wear the same clothes even if those clothes are inappropriate to the weather
- Looking at the finer detail rather than the overall picture—for example, looking at the bold outline of an image rather than what the actual image is
- Playing rigidly with toys—setting up a doll's house or a Playmobil game but not actually playing with it
- Narrow interest or extreme interest in toys or certain topics
- Rituals and compulsions about daily occurrences—for example, Mummy always reading the bedtime story or always using the same cup for a drink

When you read the preceding list, did a few behaviors seem familiar and did you start to recognize some of these traits in your own child? The stage where you've got this gut feeling about your child's development being slightly delayed and you don't know whether you should be worried or not is the hardest place for a parent. Perhaps you're thinking that there's nothing to be worried about: "They'll grow out of it," "They need more time," "I couldn't talk until I was 3 and I'm fine now," or "They're just lazy" (by the way, children are never lazy with language development—they will always be communicating to the best of their ability).

My advice is definitely not to watch and wait. Get some help sooner rather than later because this is an area where early intervention can make a world of difference, and your worry will start to subside if you have someone to help and support you. Perhaps start with your family doctor. Also take a look at the M-CHAT, a screening assessment that you can easily find online. It will help you to decipher which areas are tricky for your little one and then you can look at ways to help from my Top Tip Time section and start to implement some of my strategies right away. You will soon begin to see a positive difference.

## What causes autism?

We know that there's no single cause of autism, just as there's no single type of autism. Over the last few years, scientists have suggested that the causes of autism may be genetic, and it is most likely that multiple genes are responsible rather than a single gene. There is no evidence to suggest that autism is caused by emotional deprivation or a person's upbringing.

## At what age is autism most commonly diagnosed?

The average age for an autism diagnosis is between 3 and 4 years old. Yet many parents first become concerned at around 18 months. In fact, the latest research indicates that many children with autism show signs in their first year, when developmental delays—particularly with regard to language and communication development, the areas most associated with autism, become evident.

Some of the first traits parents may notice in their little ones are a preference for walking on tiptoes or making screeching noises while they play. They may line up their cars, flap their hands in excitement or rage, throw a major tantrum if a cookie breaks, become a fussy eater, struggle to take turns or follow the rules in a game, and so on. These would all be considered characteristics of autism.

But I always remind parents that for a child to receive a formal diagnosis of autism, they have to display a relatively large number of these characteristics and satisfy rigid criteria that health care professionals find in the DSM-5 and the World Health Organization's International Classification of Diseases, Revision 11.

# AUSTISM: SPECTRUMS ARE OUT— IT'S ALL ABOUT THE WHEEL

Most of us are aware that autism is described as "being on a spectrum"—a horizontal line that runs from people who have more traits of autism to people who have fewer traits of autism (previously referred to as "higher" or "lower" functioning autism, in which someone is positioned somewhere along this line).

In recent years, however, we've moved away from this analogy and opted for a wheel shape that has a number of sections relating to various autistic features, where each area affects someone's development at a different level of severity. It is important to identify these areas of strength and challenge so that we can implement some strategies, change the environment, and adapt our own behaviors accordingly to help and support.

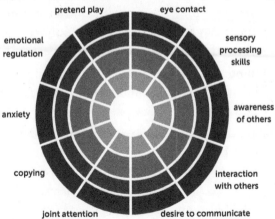

We have also thankfully moved away from the terms "high" and "low" functioning because there is an expectation that children who are high functioning should manage okay, but the reality might be very different. Some children who are considered high functioning may really struggle with shopping malls or assemblies, and therefore the high-functioning label puts pressure on the child and their family to oblige. Autism is autism— it affects every child differently and each child's individual needs should be unpacked to find the best interventions and support systems for that child.

Areas in which children with social communication difficulties or suspected autism may need help are as follows.

- **Engaging with others.** We need to help our children understand that other people can help them when it comes to play, their basic needs (food, drink, and nappy change), and comfort and support. Not only that, but other people can be fun! (Cue "The Entertainer"; see page 28. Here's your time to shine!)

- **Joint attention.** This is when two people focus on the same thing at the same time. Young children are very easily distracted, and learning to focus can be especially hard for some children. In order to thrive and learn, children have to engage with an adult at certain times for assistance, so we need to encourage our children to focus for longer.

- **Communication skills.** These are often delayed because children haven't yet understood that language can be functional and it can be used to request, comment, protest and seek information.

- **Theory of mind.** We also need to encourage children to understand that our thoughts and feelings may differ from their own, and that's okay. (See page 293.)

- **Emotional regulation.** Living in a world that is unpredictable, where even the people can be unpredictable, can create anxiety. On top of that, children who are autistic might also have sensory processing difficulties that cause a heightened or lowered ability to send sensory messages from the body to the brain about when they feel sad, excited, and so on. Consequently, their emotions are very difficult to regulate.

- **Feeling secure and safe.** This is the optimal state for learning. Children often struggle to "stay regulated" in new places or with new people, as we've mentioned, so we need to try to keep the environment as predictable as possible.

So, what can we do to help?

Let's start by unpacking these areas in more detail and, in doing so, remember that there may be a few ups and downs along the way—sometimes of roller-coaster magnitude—and you may not see results overnight, so don't give up on a strategy too quickly (like using a visual timetable, for instance). Remember, if you can't see an immediate effect, it doesn't mean you're doing something wrong; think of these early stages as planting a seed before the tree starts to grow (see pages 16–17).

## WHAT TO DO IF YOUR CHILD ISN'T INTERESTED IN ENGAGING WITH OTHERS

Remember the Language Cake in chapter 1? (See page 15.) Remember that in order for spoken language to grow, the skills on the plate of the cake need to be in place first—these are the skills for engaging with others: having a desire to communicate, listening, waiting, turn-taking, memory, attention, play (pretend play and imaginative/symbolic play), and eye contact. These are exactly the skills that young children with autism struggle with, so it is of paramount importance for the overall success with spoken language and social communication that we help and support this part of communication first.

**Top Tip Time** **Engaging with others**

- If a child needs help with their social communication skills and ability to engage with others, who better to help than . . . people themselves! Try games that involve people rather than objects. You could try peekaboo, chase, tickling, or Daddy-be-a-horsey.

- Develop play sequences (these are also known as play routines) into your child's play. This is a tricky one, but every little game has a sort of routine. Picture peekaboo; for instance: You put the cloth over your head, you say, "Where's Mummy, where's Mummy gone?," then you slowly, slowly pull the cloth off, once you meet each other's eyes, you shout "Boo!," then you say, "Again. Mummy hide," and you start the routine again. The reason for this is that once the play sequence is established, you pause so that they can contribute or even change it. Your child must communicate with you about the changes.

- Try mirror work. Most children love looking at themselves in the mirror, and this will help a child to look at you and be interested in exploring your face. Labeling parts of the face (nose, mouth, eyes) are often some of the first words a child might say or understand. Sit your child on your lap so they can see their own face and yours in a mirror and try saying some simple babble sounds over and over again—"mmm," "bbb," "ddd," and "ppp." Encourage your child to make a pointy finger and point and label all your facial features. Allow your child to take the lead.

- Try copy boxes. Copy boxes are two sets of identical toys, one set in each box. One box is presented to your child, and one you keep for yourself. (I tend to choose photocopy paper boxes for mine—they're the perfect size). The toys you choose for the boxes should be relevant to your child's developmental stage. The idea is to play with your child by getting down on their level, sitting opposite them, offering them their box, waiting to see what your child chooses and what they do with that item. Then you copy their actions, as well as their sounds and words, as they play. Don't ask questions, and use brief, simple language to describe what the child and you are doing—for example, "brushing hair," "hat on," "bang the spoon on the box," and so on. Some children may be more relaxed if you speak in a very quiet voice or not at all.

A copy box could contain the following items.

| | |
|---|---|
| 2 cars | 2 toothbrushes |
| 2 play sets of cups | 2 containers or bags |
| 2 dolls or teddies | 8 bricks |
| 2 play spoons | 2 shakers |
| 2 hairbrushes | 2 toy hammers |

| | |
|---|---|
| 2 party horns | 2 hats |
| 2 books | 2 scarves |
| 2 balls | 2 windup toys |

Look out for the following behaviors.

- Your child may look at you or show in some other way that they have noticed you are copying them—great! Keep up this momentum.

- Once the child gets used to being copied in this way, they may keep looking at what you are doing. They may look or pause in their play to wait for you to copy them. This is the beginning of turn taking; the child does something and you copy.

- When you are sure the child is aware that you are copying them, try adding something extra to the play, something similar to what the child has just done, then pause and see if they copy you.

- Last but not least: Don't put pressure on your child to talk by saying, "What's that?," "Say car," "When you say it, you can have it," and so on. This does not work. In fact, it may make your child more reluctant to speak to all. If they could say the word, they would. Your child is not lazy, they will be trying the very best they can at this particular moment in time.

Copying is a very important skill to practice as it encourages engagement and eye contact and allows the adult and child to socialize together. Copy boxes are particularly useful for children who tend to play on their own and don't easily respond to playful attention from adults or other children. It works best when you allow your child to take the lead in your play and interactions, and it provides valuable opportunities for adults to add simple language and gestures, and sometimes you might also be able to extend or develop your child's play skills.

Another well-known strategy for developing a child's ability to engage is called intensive interaction. This approach stems around copying everything a child does in a non-intrusive and subtle way.

Speech and language pathologists use it a lot, and there are tons of videos and articles about it on YouTube and Google.

# WHAT TO DO IF YOU CAN'T GET YOUR CHILD'S ATTENTION

Joint attention is when two people share an interest in the same thing at the same time. It happens when one person shares the moment with another by making eye contact, pointing, or using words and sounds to alert the other person to something they are looking at. Picture yourself sitting at a table with a box of markers and some paper. You hold the marker out for your child to take but they don't take it. So, you then make a mark on the paper and say, "Ooh look," trying to spark some interest. Still no response. Your child is perhaps too busy in their own game, perhaps they're looking around the room instead or even sitting with you but seem not to respond to your attempts to interact with them.

A child that fits this description is having difficulty with two main areas: their social interaction (not understanding what is expected from them in a given social situation) and joint attention (where an adult and a child are focusing on the same activity at the same time).

Conversely, picture a child who sees a plane, looks at their parent to get their reaction, and looks back at the plane. This child has understood the benefits of joint attention.

To be able to jointly attend, a child needs to be able to shift attention between an adult and the object that they are interested in. This can be tricky for some children. But it is so important because it builds the early social skills of enabling in a two-way interaction. It also allows the child to copy, listen to, and learn the language that the adult is using.

**Top Tip Time** Improving focus and engagement

First off, ensure you have your 10 minutes of Special Time every day where you incorporate at least one of the following strategies. Notice that very few of the following activities and strategies focus directly on saying words. They are all are about improving focus and engagement.

- Make yourself a fun person to play with! Use a lively voice, lots of facial expressions, and big gestures! Leave lots of pauses and speak in a singsongy voice that is more interesting to listen to.

- Make eye contact as easy as possible for your child—kneel, sit, or lie down so you are at the same level as they are.

- Play games that your child really enjoys—for example, singing, bubbles, and physical games to capture their attention.

- Join in with your child's play and copy what they are doing with sounds and actions. Add in extra words and comment on what they are looking at.

- Use the Say What You See strategy while they play—that is, provide a simple descriptive commentary as your child plays, putting their thought into words. Use repetitive here-and-now language. For example, while playing chase you can add a repetitive commentary—"Fast, fast, fast" or "Run, run, run," "Mummy stop," "Mummy go." Don't worry about keeping your sentences too simple—some children are attracted to the intonation patterns in short sentences and learn language by tuning in to them (this is called Gestalt Language Processing; for more information, see meaningfulspeech.com). Remember to pause to allow your child to copy the words and sounds you say. If a very chatty parent comes into the clinic, I consciously slow down my language so that they copy—it's really hard to tell a parent that they talk too fast and they're not giving their child a chance to speak!

- If your child isn't pointing yet, try to encourage finger isolation. Get some books that have textured parts; for example, say, "That's not my . . ." and hold your child's three fingers back so only one is pointing. Label the objects as you point together. Pause to see if your child looks at you. If finding the pointing shape is difficult for your child, try some finger painting or pushing your child's finger into some Play-Doh.

- Try an attention box—fill a small box with sensory-based activities such as toys that will wind up, flash, make a noise of some sort, then knock on the top on the box saying, "Knock, knock, knock, what's in the box?," then open the box and pull the toys out one by one to show your child. You can say, "more" and "bye-bye" as you take the objects in and out of the box.

- Encourage your child to move their attention between you, as in your face and your voice, and what you are both playing with. If your child really struggles to give eye contact, don't worry; joint attention can still be achieved.

- Allow your child to take the lead when you play together; for example, if a child wants to stack some puzzle pieces rather than insert them into the board, go with it, allow them, and say, "Building up, up, up," or if a child wants to turn a page before you've read the whole text, allow them. This way they will stay focused for longer.

- Get into a position where you can see exactly what your child is looking at so that you can be sure that you're modeling the right word and sound. This is particularly difficult when outdoors (but do your best)!

- Sometimes a small table and chair can help to expand your little one's attention to a task for longer. It will also help you to get down to your child's level, which assists communication.

Here are some more joint-attention activities.

- Roll a ball/car down a ramp or throw a ball back and forth.

- Do a jigsaw puzzle together.
- Sing songs with actions, like "Row, Row, Row Your Boat."
- Hold hands and dance to your child's favorite song.
- Hold a sheet or blanket with your child and rock a baby doll.
- Blow bubbles.
- Play peekaboo or hide-and-seek with toys.
- Blow up balloons and let them go to fly around the room.
- Play physical games such as chase and tickles or Daddy-be-a-horsey.
- Build towers and knock them down.

## WHAT TO DO IF YOUR CHILD STRUGGLES WITH COMMUNICATION SKILLS

Once your child has started to understand that engaging with others and sharing joint attention can be rewarding and even fun, their communication skills will start to grow. As you know, we speech therapists accept all methods of communication, be it a gesture, a cry, a reach, an eye-point (looking at what they want), echolalia, giving a picture or using a device—even avoidance, pushing, and hitting are forms of communication. Basically, all behavior is considered communication. So let's try a few "communications temptations" to get started. Remember, any of the forms of communication previously listed can be accepted as responses. The key is *not* to let your child get frustrated, as this type of negative interaction will be unappealing for your child's wanting to repeat it and is therefore counterproductive. Here are some examples to try.

**Top Tip Time** **Tempting your children to communicate**

- You know your child wants to go out. Put your hand on the handle, don't open it, and wait for your child to communicate with you to ask you to open it. This may be a look at you, a look at the door and then look at you, or your child might put your hand on the handle or jerk their body forward meaning "do it." Once you notice that attempt to communicate, say, "Open the door." Remember to use your singsongy phrase to make the sentence more attractive to copy.

- On a swing, pull the swing back and encourage your little one to communicate with you to let the swing go. Do this over and over again. This may be a kick of their feet or a look.

- Pretend you don't know what they want when they go to the fridge. See how much they can communicate with you but remember not to let them get frustrated, turning a positive interaction into a negative one. There is a fine line here, and you, the parent, will know best how far you can go before your child feels frustrated. Communication has to be positive, so if you are frequently pushing or allowing frustration to creep in, this will be counterproductive and create negativity about learning to communicate or an avoidance in wanting to communicate at all.

- Give your child something they want but put it in a see-through container with a sealed lid. They will have to communicate to you what they want before you open the container. You could try sticking a line of pictures on a few see-through containers. The pictures would be "Mummy" (a picture of your face), "open" (a picture of your hand opening, which is the sign language), "box" (a box with an open lid). Change the picture of your face to Daddy or a teacher's name: "Miss Stenner," "open," "the box," or "Daddy" "open," "the box," etc.

- During snack time, give a couple of raisins or chips to tempt them, and wait for your child to request that they want more. A request for more could be looking or giving the bowl to you to fill it up. It doesn't have to be words.

- During ready-steady-go games, don't do the action expected on the word "go" and see what your child does to request you to do it.

- Start to sing a familiar song and stop in the middle of a lyric. Will your child communicate to encourage you to carry on?

- Do something "wrong," like put a funny wig or hat on, put a shoe on before a sock, a glove on a foot, etc. Will your child react? Will they communicate this reaction to you?

- Hand a deflated balloon to your child or the bubble dipper and see how they communicate what they want.

- Present your child with part of an activity—for instance, paint without the brush, toothbrush without the paste, yogurt without the spoon, paper without the paper, bubbles with the lid on, etc.

- Put a really motivating object in your hand and wait for your child to say that they want it.

Here are other activities to try.

- Exploit every opportunity to bring repetitive words and phrases into daytime routines and games—for example, when your child lifts their hand up to be picked up, say "Up, up" and wait for a response; at snack time, "Wash, wash, wash your hands"; when you go out, "Coat on, shoes on, oooooopen the door"; when you get into the car, "Open the door, in your seat, strap on, click," etc. You can try accompanying the words to a familiar tune or melody because words are retained better in your brain when they are accompanied by a tune. The "Skip to My Lou" tune always seems to work well! This is a known music therapy technique. It's called "Melodic Intonation Therapy," and it works well for children when there is a query about autism.

- You could try using a plastic echo microphone to encourage your child to copy the noises and the words you say. This can be very motivating for a young child.

- If your child is keen on screen time, one of my favorite apps for young children is called "Special Words." It has a set of core pictures, and the child has to match a picture to a picture, then a word to a word, and then a word to a picture. You can add your own pictures of your child's favorite people, and when you get it right it cheers, which the children love.

- You may have noticed that people who have autism-like systems; we already mentioned that desire for sameness and predictability. Well, autistic children often like letters and numbers, which are predictable and orderly. So, let's use these to motivate our children to use functional language. If your child wants you to count, encourage them to say, "Mummy count," "Granddad count," or "More counting please."

- Some children really struggle with spoken communication, and if this is the case, we need to try a device, such as an iPad, or pictures instead. Pictures are used in a multitude of ways for autistic children: now and next boards, visual timetables, PECS (Picture Exchange Communication System), labels for toys and toy boxes (making them predictable), social storybooks, etc. Parents can get worried when SLPs mention a device or pictures because they fear we are moving away from encouraging actual words but enhancing all forms of motivating ways to communicate can only be a bonus, so go with it.

- Model appropriate conversation and social skills—for example, social greetings, body language, personal space, asking for help, starting and maintaining conversation.

- Use comic strip conversations: They are simple visual representations of conversations and can show the things that are actually said in a conversation, how people might be feeling, and what people's intentions might be. Use comic strip conversations with stick figures and symbols to represent social interactions and abstract aspects of conversation, and use colors to represent the emotional content of a statement or message.

Although teaching direct social skills such as eye contact, body language, topic starters, and topic maintenance is a little controversial (because we should be encouraging our children to learn the skill of accepting all different styles of social communication), your child might require specific social skills and life-skills teaching to guide and support their initiations and responses to different situations, especially if they are feeling anxious about this.

# WHAT TO DO IF YOUR CHILD STRUGGLES TO UNDERSTAND THAT OTHER PEOPLE HAVE DIFFFERENT THOUGHTS FROM THEIR OWN

True theory of mind doesn't establish itself in children until they reach 4 or 5 years old and can only be mastered when children have developed the skills for joint attention, intentionality (understanding that others' actions are goal-directed and arise out of unique beliefs and desires), and imitation.

As this book is primarily aimed at parents of children under 4 years old, your little one may be a bit young to develop this skill. For the future though, the best resources I have used to develop theory of mind are the social-thinking resources. These encourage children to understand that every person has a brain for thinking thoughts and a heart for feeling feelings. Whatever life throws at us, from death through to broken crackers, every person will have a thought in their brain and feeling in their heart that will differ from one's own. Another way of describing this is "mind-blindness," similar to color-blindness but for the brain's thoughts and feelings. And you'll find that once this concept becomes better established—that your child establishes the ability to see things from another person's point of view—life becomes a little easier for you and your whole family.

# WHAT TO DO IF YOUR CHILD STRUGGLES WITH EMOTIONAL REGULATION

Children on with autism tend to struggle to keep their emotions regulated. They may overreact or underreact to situations they're confronted with. Again, little children are all prone to this, but when it becomes a problem and interferes with everyday life and activities, it's time to think about how you can help. Here are some suggestions.

**Top Tip Time**  **Helping your child to regulate their emotions across the day**

- Always label your child's feelings and emotions as and when they experience them. So, when your little one screams because they don't want to go in the car seat say, "You're feeling cross with Mummy because you don't want to go in your seat, but all children going swimming must sit in their seat." When they bounce up and down because Granny is arriving shortly, say, "You're excited. Granny is coming soon."

- Simplify and lower your language level. Your child will benefit from those around them pitching their model of language at the right level for them to learn. This is particularly important when your child is emotional, such as angry, frustrated, tired, or upset. Our ability to interpret language decreases during emotional extremes and overloading with language can make situations or behavior worse. Allow time to calm before discussing incidents or consider using a nonverbal, visual approach, which reduces the cognitive load.

- Actively preplan your events. If you need to, you can role-play situations that are about to occur using small figurines.

- Provide visual supports such as visual timetables, now and next boards, and task-management plans (breaking tasks, such as going to the bathroom, down into tiny little steps using pictures). Create a safe space where your child can practice these skills with their peers, in a small corner of the classroom or in a small group of children, for example. Remember, using visuals throughout the day will be very helpful to keep your child regulated, especially in transitions from one place to another or one activity to another—which can be very stressful for children who need predictability in order to feel safe and secure. The benefits of using visuals are obvious; they're permeant, they enable processing time, they help prepare children for the next task/transition, they help children to *see* what you mean, and you can take a visual wherever you go so they build independence and reduce anxiety. A multitude of companies have photo or symbol libraries, or parents can use Google Images.

- Praise and provide specific feedback when your child has shown good skills. "Well done" or "good job" don't help them to know what they are doing well.

- Encourage flexible thinking. Be a good role model and become a flexible thinker yourself. Don't always insist on doing the same things the same way every day: Think up new rules for your favorite games; for example, Connect 4 can become Connect 6. Think of new ways to do everyday experiences. Can you walk a new way to the store or to school? When supporting your child to solve a problem, have them think of three solutions before they decide on the best option.

- Use Social Behavior Mapping to teach about the specific relationship between behaviors, others' perspectives, others' actions (consequences) and your child's own emotions about those around them.

- Build calm or movement breaks into your day so that your child can learn to regulate their emotions. In a nutshell, if *you* are anxious, seek help and support for yourself, too!

- Encourage your child to examine their thoughts and consider how accurate and realistic they are.

- Encourage your child to talk to you about things they are struggling with.

- Provide positive feedback when they communicate when there is a problem, and work toward a good solution.

- Co-regulate with your child. Understand that if your emotions throughout the day are like a roller coaster, so will your child's. For example, if there's a surprise guest coming to nursery later, and you continuously talk about it in a hyperexcited way, your child will follow suit and remain in a heightened state of alertness the whole day, too.

- Learn to identify what triggers your child's emotions and try to detect a pattern.

# WHAT TO DO IF YOUR CHILD STRUGGLES TO FEEL SAFE AND SECURE

Boosting your child's self-esteem sounds so easy, but sometimes it can be a real struggle, especially with children who sometimes feel they don't fit in, or perhaps can't articulate that this is how they feel but can sense it subconsciously. They might even be able to sense that their parents are worried about them, and these factors combined can really affect their self-esteem. Use these tips to bolster their confidence and ensure that your child feels safe and secure.

**Top Tip Time** **Helping your child to feel safe and secure**

- Make your day as predictable as possible. Use "objects of reference" to help signify what is about to happen. Bring a familiar bib to your child when it's time for eating. Show your child a rubber duck when it's bath time and use the duck in the bath. Use photos of the swimming pool or caregiver to help your child understand what is about to happen. Sing the same songs when you are about to do a particular activity so that your child won't feel alarmed. For example, "We're going in the car, we're going in the car, hi-ho the merry-oh, we're going in the car" (to the tune of "The Farmer in the Dell").

- Give clear and direct instructions. Avoid using ambiguous or complicated instructions because your child will find it difficult to process and interpret these. Be direct and give instructions in the order that your child needs to do them. Avoid indirect directions such as "Everybody needs to be sitting down," as your child may not understand that this instruction includes them. Be specific and direct the instruction at your child by using their name.

- Avoid ambiguous or nonliteral language because your child can find it difficult to understand what it means. Two examples are "It's raining buckets outside" and "Have you fallen out?" It's difficult to avoid this type of language but make sure that you clearly explain what this means.

- Create structure during unstructured times. Your child might find it more difficult when there is no clear structure, purpose, or routine such as free play at nursery. Consider giving your little one a specific role at break time or lunchtime. Give clear boundaries about what will and will not be tolerated.

- Use your child's interests and experiences to help them understand different contexts. Try to relate what they see in books or what they learn to real-life situations as often as possible.

- Encourage a growth mindset. Praise your child for their effort rather than their talent.

- When you face challenges or make mistakes, model a positive attitude and explain how you'll try and try again.

- Explain that making mistakes is okay; everyone makes mistakes . . . it's how we learn. No one can be the best at everything and that's okay.

- Encourage your child to try new things and praise them for trying new things.

- Remember to "Take 10"—your 10 minutes of Special Time every day is integral to talk, laugh, and do something fun together that will make your child feel special.

## UNDERSTANDING SENSORY PROCESSING DISORDER

Researchers have found that a child's sensory processing skills and their ability to integrate their senses have a huge impact on a child's ability to stay calm and focused. Children with autism may have a heightened or lowered reaction to sensory stimuli or difficulty integrating their senses (known as sensory processing disorder) so you should be aware of noises, tastes, textures, touch, smells, and sights in the environment that could be triggers for distress for your child. These might include the smell of your laundry detergent or coffee machine, clothes labels, scratchy or rough fabrics, or even heavy seams and pockets, multiple textures on one plate of food (let your child feel what they are eating so that they can get as much sensory information from it as possible), high-pitched buzzes from the TV, noises from central heating pipes, or the sun shining in their face.

Did you know that we actually have eight senses that receive information from our daily experiences and send information to our brain to enable us to process it?

We have five senses that are external senses—touch, taste, smell, hearing, vision—but we also have three internal senses: vestibular, proprioceptive, and interoceptive.

- **The vestibular sense allows your body to sense when you are moving.** You might see a child constantly on the go or simply rocking their body to help them feel calm and focused.

- **The proprioceptive sense enables you to understand where your body is in space.** So, if I lift my arm, signals from my muscles and joints are being sent to my brain to tell it what my arm is doing. Perhaps you have seen a child jumping or flapping their hands (this can sometimes be referred to as "stimming"). This child is stimulating the proprioceptive sense and often needs deep pressure massage to help the senses send the signals to the brain.

- **The interoceptive sense is the internal body feeling—for example, hunger, thirst, pain, too hot or too cold, tired, nervous (butterflies in your tummy).** Have you ever seen a child wearing a T-shirt in the middle of winter or perhaps you think a child is overreacting when they're hungry—but the child hasn't sensed those feelings until they are starving or absolutely freezing cold? Because of this, a child with interoceptive difficulty can be misconstrued as having bad behavior.

Unless your child's sensory system—and sensory processing skills—is well integrated, and functioning well, they will be easily distracted by all the sensory information around them. If your child is struggling to focus and isn't improving over time, I encourage you to seek the support of a sensory integration trained occupational therapist (OT). There are two other factors that have a HUGE impact on a child's ability to focus: hearing and sleep. Can your child actually hear? If you're not sure, ask your doctor for a referral to audiology to check your child's hearing; hearing and listening are two completely different skills. And if a child isn't getting enough sleep, this will have a profound impact on your child's ability to listen and focus. Look at your child's sleep skills and seek help from your doctor if you think this is a factor.

Last but not least, you are your child's best role model for good listening. If a child is valued, respected, and made to feel important by an adult who listens to them, you will become their role model, and they will try as hard as they possibly can to listen and respect you while you're talking, too.

If you've started to think that your little one may have autism, there's a lot that can be done to help and a lot of support out there to receive. The main message is to focus on what motivates your child and to adapt their environment to help them learn. It can sometimes feel daunting, but step by step you'll see progress being made.

# A Final Word from Me

I've really enjoyed writing this book and sharing my expertise with you. I hope you've found our journey from babbling babies to talking tots entertaining and inspiring and that I've filled you with confidence when it comes to communicating with your child. If my Top Tip Time games have given you lots of laughter and brought some fun to those afternoons when you just don't know how to entertain your little one, then I've achieved what I set out to do. I'd be even more delighted if I knew that every reader had used Say What You See, stayed one step ahead, and ditched the dummy!

As I've said all along, you are your child's best resource for learning, so keep entertaining, educating, and inspiring your little one, and feel confident in the fact that you are giving your child the very best possible start in life. Good luck!

## DEVELOPMENTAL MILESTONES FROM 0 TO 48 MONTHS

These milestones marked with an asterisk (*) have been provided by the website speechandlanguage.org.uk and are reproduced with kind permission.

### Speech and language development milestones: 0–6 months

Here is a set of milestones for speech and language development to be used as a guide for parents. As I keep saying, all children develop skills at different rates, but by six months, usually a child will

- turn toward a sound when they hear it,
- be startled by loud noises,
- watch your face when you talk to them,
- recognize your voice,
- smile and laugh when other people smile and laugh,
- make sounds to themselves, such as coos, gurgles, and babbling sounds.
- make noises, like coos or squeals, to get your attention, and
- use different cries to express different needs (for example, one cry to signify hunger, another to indicate tiredness, and so on).

## Speech and language development milestones: 6–12 months

Children develop skills at different rates but, by one year, usually a child will

- listen carefully and turn to someone talking on the other side of the room,
- look at you when you speak and when their name is called,
- babble strings of sounds, such as "no-no" and "go-go,"
- make noises, point, and look at you to get your attention,
- smile at people who are smiling at them,
- start to understand words like "bye-bye" and "up," especially when a gesture is used at the same time,
- recognize the names of familiar objects or people such as "car" and "Daddy,"
- enjoy action songs and rhymes and get excited when sung to, and
- take turns in conversations, babbling back to an adult.

## Speech and language development milestones: 18–24 months

Children develop skills at different rates but, by 24 months, usually children will

- concentrate on activities for longer, like playing with a particular toy,
- sit and listen to simple stories with pictures,
- understand between 200 and 500 words,
- understand more simple questions and instructions—for example, "Where is your shoe?" and "Show me your nose,"
- copy sounds and words a lot,
- use 50 or more single words. These will also become more recognizable to those not familiar with the child,
- start to put short sentences together with two to three words, such as "More juice" or "Bye, Nanny,"
- enjoy pretend play with their toys, such as feeding dolly, and
- use a limited number of sounds in words—often these are "p," "b," "t," "d," "m," and "w." Children will also often drop the end sound or syllable off words at this stage. They can usually be understood about half of the time.

## Speech and language development milestones: 24–36 months

Children develop skills at different rates but, by age 3, usually a child will

- listen to and remember simple stories with pictures,
- understand longer instructions, such as "Make Teddy jump" or "Where's Mummy's coat?,"
- understand simple "who," "what," and "where" questions,
- use up to 300 words,
- put 4 or 5 words together to make short sentences, such as "Want more red juice" or "He took my ball,"

- ask lots of questions—they will want to find out the names of things and learn new words,
- use verbs (action words, such as "run" and "fall") as well as nouns (naming words),
- start to use simple plurals by adding "s,"—for example, "shoes" or "cars,"
- use a wider range of speech sounds. However, many children will shorten longer words, such as saying "nana" instead of "banana." They may also have difficulty where lots of sounds happen together in a word (e.g., they may say "pider" instead of "spider"),
- often have problems saying more difficult sounds, like "sh," "ch," "th," and "r." However, people who know them can mostly understand them,
- now play more with other children and share things, and
- sometimes sound as if they are stuttering. They are usually trying to share their ideas before their language skills are ready. This is perfectly normal. Just show you are listening and allow plenty of time for your child to speak.

## Speech and language development milestones: 36–48 months

Children develop skills at different rates but, by age 4, usually a child will

- listen to longer stories and answer questions about a storybook they have just read,
- understand and often use color, number and time-related words; for example, "red car," "three fingers" and "yesterday/tomorrow,"
- be able to answer questions about why something has happened (in the past tense),
- use longer sentences and link sentences together,
- describe events that have already happened—for instance, "We went park,"

- enjoy make-believe play,
- start to like simple jokes,
- ask many questions using words like "what," "where," and "why,"
- still make mistakes with tenses, such as saying "runned" for "ran" and "swimmed" for "swam,"
- have difficulties with a small number of sounds—for example "r," "w," "l," "f," "th," "sh," "ch," "j," and "dz," and
- start to be able to plan games with others.

# Glossary

**anticipation game**—a game in which the adult will expect the child to do something to take part in the game

**articulators**—the jaw, lips, and tongue

**attention/listening**—the ability to focus attention on the person talking to receive an intricate message

**auditory memory**—the ability to process, analyze, and recall orally presented information

**babble phase**—the stage where babies are experimenting with consonant sounds but not yet using recognizable words

**blends or consonant clusters**—when two consonant sounds appear together (e.g., train)

**comprehension**—understanding what spoken words mean

**concentration**—the ability to focus on a given activity for an appropriate amount of time in order to complete a task

**concept**—an idea, a thought, or a notion that corresponds to a class of entities (e.g., big, small, medium)

**container play**—a game of transferring objects from one container to another, enjoyed by children of approximately 2 to 2½ years

**conversational babble**—when the babble becomes more elaborate, reaching four or five syllables, and varied tones are used, such as "goo-eee-yah," "bay-me-ooo-du," "ka-da-bu-ba" (usually appears by about 10 months)

**delay**—when a child's language is developing in the right sequence but at a slower rate

**difficulty/impairment**—a difficulty is something that may be overcome; an impairment is something thought to be longer term.

**disorder**—when language is not typical of normal language development. Children will have some language skills but not others, or the way in which these skills develop will be different than usual.

**dysphagia**—an inability or partial inability to swallow

**expressive language**—the use of words and sentences to communicate needs, wants, and thoughts

**gesture**—the natural use of hands or body to communicate in order to emphasize a point (e.g., palms facing upward accompanied by a shoulder shrug for "I don't know")

**grammar**—how words combine to form sentences

**jargon**—speech therapy term for conversational babble

**key word**—a word that your child has to understand in order to carry out an instruction

**language**—the combination of sounds, words, and sentences used to express meaning

**minimal pair**—pairs of words that only differ in one phonological element (e.g., "Kate" and "gate")

**motherese/parentese**—a unique form of speech used by adults when talking to babies, also known as child-directed or infant-directed speech and baby-talk

**phonics**—a method of teaching letters using their speech sounds in preparation for reading and spelling (e.g., the "s" sound would be "sss" not "suh" or "ess")

**phonology**—the way a child uses individual speech sounds to formulate words

**play-based learning**—using play to encourage learning

**pre-babble**—the sounds that are made unintentionally before babble appears, including vowel sounds and experimental noises

**pretend play**—using props in an imaginative way such as role-play (e.g., the home corner or a shoe store)

**pre-verbal stage**—the stage before a child uses words to communicate. Infancy is, by definition, a pre-verbal phase in development. (The Latin word *infans* means "without language.")

**reduplicated babble**—when the same sound is repeated in babble (e.g., "ba-ba" or "goo-goo")

**signs**—using your hands to convey meaning in a formal way

**SLP**—speech-language pathologist (or speech therapist)

**small world play**—playing with miniature toys that represent real life (e.g., a doll's house and furniture)

**speech sounds**—sounds that are used within a given language

**symbolic play**—pretending that one object represents another (e.g., a colander as a helmet)

**symbols**—pictures that represent meaning (e.g., the sign for an accessible bathroom)

**tongue thrust**—a reflex that causes tongue protrusion that prevents choking, which should disappear by 4 to 6 months

**variegated babble**—the second stage of babbling, which involves putting two different consonant sounds together, such as "mu-bu" or "du-wu," which should appear by about 8 to 9 months

**vocabulary**—the total number of words a person knows and uses

**word**—a consistently spoken utterance that represents a particular object or person

# Notes

## Introduction

1  B. Hart and T. R. Risley, *Meaningful Differences in the Everyday Experience of Young American Children* (Baltimore: Paul H. Brookes Publishing Co., 1995).

## Chapter 1

1  "Recognizing a Problem" was adapted by Karen Fern (Oxfordshire Children's SLT) and Susie Fuller (EYSENIT), with kind permission from I CAN (ican.org.uk).

2  J. C. O'Kane and J. Goldbart, *Communication Before Speech—Development and Assessment*, 2nd ed. (London: David Fulton, 1998).

3  The descriptions of parent types have been adapted from the book *It Takes Two to Talk: A Practical Guide for Parents of Children with Language Delays* (Pepper and Weitzman, 2004). A Hanen Center publication. Reprinted with permission.

## Chapter 2

1  A. Blasi et al., "Early Specialization for Voice and Emotion Processing in the Infant Brain," *Current Biology* 21, no. 14 (June 2011): 1220–24.

2  M. S. Zeedyk, in collaboration with the National Literacy Trust and the Sutton Trust, "The Impact of Stroller Orientation on Parent–Infant Interaction and Infant Stress," 2007.

3  E. D. Thiessen, E. A. Hill, and J. R. Saffran, "Infant-Directed Speech Facilitates Word Segmentation," *Infancy* 7 (January 1, 2005): 49–67.

## Chapter 3

1  Adapted from the National Autistic Society's EarlyBird Programme Parent Book (autism.org.uk/earlybird).

2  D. Lewkowicz, "Babies Lip-Read Before Talking," *Science News* 181, no. 3 (February 2012): 9.

3  C. J. Limb, "Structural and Functional Neural Correlates of Music Perception," *The Anatomical Record* 288A, no. 4 (April 2006).

4  K. J. Topping, R. Dekhinet, and S. Zeedyk, "Hindrances for Parents in Enhancing Child Language," *Educational Psychology Review* 23, no. 3 (September 2011): 413–55.

5  L. Camaioni, F. Bellagamba, and A. Fogel, "A Longitudinal Examination of the Transition to Symbolic Communication in the Second Year of Life," *Infant and Child Development* 12, no. 2 (June 2003): 177–95.

## Chapter 4

1  D. Roy, R. Patel, P. DeCamp, R. Kubat, M. Fleischman, B. Roy, N. Mavridis, S. Tellex, A. Salata, J. Guinness, M. Levit, P. Gorniak, "The Human Speechome Project," Cognitive Machines Group, MIT Media Laboratory. Presented at the 28th annual conference of the Cognitive Science Society, July 2006.

2  B. Wells and J. Stackhouse, *Children's Speech and Literacy Difficulties: A Psycholinguistic Framework* (Chichester, England: Wiley Blackwell, 1997).

## Chapter 5

1  L. Rescorla, A. Alley, and J. B. Christine, "Word Frequencies in Toddlers' Lexicons," *Journal of Speech, Language, and Hearing Research* 44 (2001): 598–609.

## Chapter 11

1  A. W. Kummer, "Ankyloglossia: To Clip or Not to Clip? That's the Question," *The ASHA Leader*, December 27, 2005.

2  Ibid.

3  M. E. Graham, "What Is Tongue Tie?," *JAMA Otolaryngology–Head & Neck Surgery* 148, no. 5 (2022): 496.

4  B. A. Lewis and L. A. Thompson, "A Study of Developmental Speech and Language Disorders in Twins," *Journal of Speech and Hearing Research* 35 (1992): 1086–94.

5  J. Cooper et al., Helping Language Development: *A Developmental Programme for Children with Early Language Handicaps* (London: Edward Arnold, 1978).

6  A. Garcia-Sierra, M. Rivera-Gaxiola, C. R. Percaccio, B. T. Conboy, H. Romo, L. Klarman, S. Ortiz, and P. K. Kuhl, "Bilingual Language Learning: An ERP Study Relating Early Brain Responses to Speech, Language Input, and Later Word Production," *Journal of Phonetics* 39, no. 4 (October 2011): 546–57.

7  J. O. Klein and S. Pelton, "Management of Otitis Media with Effusion Serous Otitis Media) in Children," UpToDate.com, accessed February 14, 2014.

# Support Groups and Organisations

**Afasic** (UK-wide parent support group) – visit www.afasic.org.uk for details of information and activities across the four countries

**British Stammering Association** – www.stamma.org

**Hanen** (programmes, resources and workshops for parents and professionals) – www.hanen.org

**Help With Talking** (independent speech and language therapy website) – www.helpwithtalking.com

**National Autistic Society** – www.autism.org.uk

**Royal College of Speech and Language Therapists** – www.rcslt.org

**Selective Mutism** parental support – www.selectivemutism.org.uk

**Speech and Language UK** (resources, information and training on children's communication development and SLCN for parents, carers and professionals) – www.speechandlanguage.org.uk

**The Owl Centre** (Assessment and Therapy services across the UK) – www.theowltherapycentre.co.uk

# Recommended Reading

## Books for Parents

*A First Language* by Roger Brown

*Baby-Led Weaning* by Gill Rapley and Tracey Murkett

*It Takes Two to Talk* by Jan Pepper and Elaine Weitzman, published by the Hanen Center

*Baby Signs* by Joy Allen

*Raising Boys: Why Boys Are Different—and How to Help Them Become Happy and Well-Balanced Men* by Steve Biddulph

*Time to Talk: Parents' Accounts of Children's Speech Difficulties* by Margaret Glogowska

*Why Love Matters* by Sue Gerhardt

## Books for Children

*At the Park* by Nicola Lathey

*Bedtime* by Nicola Lathey

*Brown Bear, Brown Bear, What Do You See?* by Bill Martin Jr. and Eric Carle

*Charlie Cook's Favorite Book* and *A Squash and a Squeeze* by Julia Donaldson and Axel Scheffler

*Chocolate Mousse for Greedy Goose* by Julia Donaldson and Nick Sharratt

*Dear Zoo* by Rod Campbell

*Funny Face* by Nicola Smee

*Handa's Surprise* by Eileen Browne

*How to Catch a Star* by Oliver Jeffers

*Hug* by Jez Alborough

## Recommended Reading

*Mixed Up Fairy Tales* by Hilary Robinson and Nick Sharratt

*Owl Babies* by Martin Waddell and Patrick Benson

*Peace at Last* by Jill Murphy

*Q Pootle 5* by Nick Butterworth

*Richard Scarry's Best First Book Ever!* by Richard Scarry

*Rosie's Walk* by Pat Hutchins

*Say Boo!* by Lynda Graham-Barber

*Spot's Opposites* by Eric Hill

*That's Not My . . .* series by Fiona Watt and Rachel Wells

*The Astonishing Secret of Awesome Man* by Michael Chabon and Jake Parker

*The Baby's Catalogue* by Janet and Allan Ahlberg

*The Gruffalo* by Julia Donaldson and Axel Scheffler

*The Gruffalo's Child* by Julia Donaldson and Axel Scheffler

*The Red Book* by Barbara Lehman

*The Spiffiest Giant in Town* by Julia Donaldson and Axel Scheffler

*The Snowman* by Raymond Briggs

*The Tickle Book* (with pop-up surprises) by Ian Whybrow and Axel Scheffler

*The Tiger Who Came to Tea* by Judith Kerr

*The Very Hungry Caterpillar* by Eric Carle

*What's the Time, Mr. Wolf?* by Annie Kubler

*We're Going on a Bear Hunt* by Michael Rosen and Helen Oxenbury

*Where's Spot?* by Eric Hill

*Where's Waldo?* by Martin Handford

*Who Sank the Boat?* by Pamela Allen

*Window* by Jeannie Baker

# Resources

## RECOMMENDED RESOURCES

- A doll, teddy bear, blocks, balls, and cars
- Babble bag
- Bubbles
- Bumbo seat
- Chewy Tube—Amazon
- Doctor's kit
- Ella's Kitchen pouches
- Fishing game
- Flash cards of everyday objects, verbs, and position words
- Photos of family members
- Sequence Rummy Challenge Cards
- What's Next? sequencing puzzle

## GENERAL GAMES FOUND IN ANY SPEECH AND LANGUAGE CLINIC

- Bowling pin set
- Flash cards
- Little furniture
- Mailbox made from an old shoebox
- Mirror
- Opposites cards
- Oral motor toy

- Pop-Up Pirate
- Pretend food and tea set
- Puppets
- Sequencing cards
- Shark attack
- Shopping game
- Small world people and animals
- Story-building jigsaw puzzle
- Z-vibe—a tool for desensitizing the mouth

Scan this code or go to bit.ly/Songs4Speech for songs that will help your child master the trickiest speech sounds.

# Index

# About the Authors

**NICOLA LATHEY** is a children's speech and language therapist specializing in children under five. She is the founder of The Owl Centre, a nationwide, multidisciplinary team of 600 clinicians founded in Oxford, England.

Originally from West Wales, she now lives in Oxford with her husband and their daughter, Jess. Nicola qualified from University College London in 1999 and, before setting up her private practice, worked for the National Health Service and abroad in Australia, Sri Lanka, and Vietnam. She was inspired to become a speech and language therapist after observing the therapy given to her younger brother with Down syndrome. This gave her a direct insight into the value of therapeutic intervention.

Nicola is a member of ASLTIP (Association of Speech and Language Therapists in Independent Practice), the Royal College of Speech and Language Therapists, and the Health Professional Council.

**TRACEY BLAKE** is an experienced journalist and editor. She has worked at the *Daily Mail* since 2005 and writes a baby blog called Small Talk on dailymail.co.uk. She lives in Buckinghamshire, England, with her partner, James, and their children, Minnie and Monty.

Tracey came up with the idea to write this book after Nicola visited her house for a social gathering. Nicola pointed out that Minnie, who was only 10 weeks old at the time, was very chatty. This surprised Tracey, as she had no idea that the sounds Minnie was making were in any way conversational.

A few months later, Nicola visited again and told Tracey that Minnie had started "babbling" (making consonant noises). Fascinated, Tracey looked for a book on how communication develops in babies, but there wasn't one. So, she called Nicola and said that they should write one together—and the rest, as they say, is history!